Second Edition

Case Studies Through the Health Care Continuum

A Workbook for the Occupational Therapy Student

Second Edition

Case Studies Through the Health Care Continuum

A Workbook for the Occupational Therapy Student

NANCY A. LOWENSTEIN, MS, OTR, BCPR
CLINICAL ASSOCIATE PROFESSOR
BOSTON UNIVERSITY COLLEGE OF HEALTH & REHABILITATION SCIENCES: SARGENT COLLEGE
BOSTON, MASSACHUSETTS

PATRICIA HALLORAN, MBA, MA, OTR/L

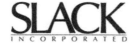

SLACK
INCORPORATED

www.Healio.com/books

ISBN: 978-1-61711-833-3

Copyright © 2015 by SLACK Incorporated

All illustrations by Janet Meade.

The procedures and practices described in this publication should be implemented in a manner consistent with the professional standards set for the circumstances that apply in each specific situation. Every effort has been made to confirm the accuracy of the information presented and to correctly relate generally accepted practices. The authors, editors, and publisher cannot accept responsibility for errors or exclusions or for the outcome of the material presented herein. There is no expressed or implied warranty of this book or information imparted by it. Care has been taken to ensure that drug selection and dosages are in accordance with currently accepted/recommended practice. Off-label uses of drugs may be discussed. Due to continuing research, changes in government policy and regulations, and various effects of drug reactions and interactions, it is recommended that the reader carefully review all materials and literature provided for each drug, especially those that are new or not frequently used. Some drugs or devices in this publication have clearance for use in a restricted research setting by the Food and Drug and Administration (FDA). Each professional should determine the FDA status of any drug or device prior to use in his or her practice.

Any review or mention of specific companies or products is not intended as an endorsement by the author or publisher.

SLACK Incorporated uses a review process to evaluate submitted material. Prior to publication, educators or clinicians provide important feedback on the content that we publish. We welcome feedback on this work.

Published by: SLACK Incorporated
                    6900 Grove Road
                    Thorofare, NJ 08086 USA
                    Telephone: 856-848-1000
                    Fax: 856-848-6091
                    www.Healio.com/books

Contact SLACK Incorporated for more information about other books in this field or about the availability of our books from distributors outside the United States.

Library of Congress Cataloging-in-Publication Data

Lowenstein, Nancy A., author.
  Case studies through the health care continuum : a workbook for the occupational therapy student / Nancy A. Lowenstein, Patricia Halloran. -- Second edition.
       p. ; cm.
  Includes index.
  Author's names reversed on the first edition.
  ISBN 978-1-61711-833-3 (alk. paper)
  I. Halloran, Patricia, author. II. Title.
  [DNLM: 1. Occupational Therapy--Case Reports. WB 555]
  RM735.45
  615.8'515--dc23
                          2015008650

Printed in the United States of America.

Last digit is print number: 10 9 8 7 6 5 4 3 2 1

DEDICATION

This book is dedicated to my students—past, present, and future. Your ability to think on your feet, analyze situations, and use theory and evidence are the basis of good practice. Keep learning and growing throughout your careers.

—*Nancy A. Lowenstein, MS, OTR, BCPR*

Contents

ACKNOWLEDGMENTS

I thank all the clients who have taught me so much over the years. Additionally, thank you to the new authors who contributed to this book. Iris Leigh, a wonderful colleague at Boston University; Cathie Marqusee, who started her occupational therapy career with me as a student; Debbie Sharp for her contributions to the pediatric cases; and Kimberly Witkowski and Katie Prizio for their contributions to the adult cases. Special thanks to Sue Gelfman who started me on my academic career, which has been the impetus for this book. An additional thank you to Allison Boris for her help with Chapter 32.

—*Nancy A. Lowenstein, MS, OTR, BCPR*

ABOUT THE AUTHORS

Nancy A. Lowenstein, MS, OTR, BCPR, is a Clinical Associate Professor at Boston University College of Health & Rehabilitation Sciences: Sargent College Occupational Therapy Entry-Level Master's Program. She has been an occupational therapist since 1987, working in the area of adult physical rehabilitation, with a specialty in multiple sclerosis. Ms. Lowenstein is currently certified by the American Occupational Therapy Association in physical rehabilitation. She is the author of *Fighting Fatigue in Multiple Sclerosis* (2009). Ms. Lowenstein has a bachelor's degree in psychology from Washington University in St. Louis, a master of arts degree in art therapy from University of Louisville, and a master of science degree from Boston University.

Patricia Halloran, MBA, MA, OTR/L, is an educator and occupational therapist. She graduated from Quinnipiac College with a bachelor of science degree in occupational therapy and holds a master of arts in applied linguistics from University of Massachusetts Boston and a master of business administration from Anna Maria College. Ms. Halloran has worked as an occupational therapist and instructor in the areas of psychiatric and physical rehabilitation, community health, and deaf education. She is currently working as a school-based occupational therapist and a special education teacher.

Contributing Authors

Susan Gelfman, MS, OTR/L, is an occupational therapist at Visions of Independence, a private practice serving elderly low-vision clients in their homes. She worked for many years at the Partial Hospital Program at Massachusetts Mental Health Center in Boston, Massachusetts.

Iris G. Leigh, CAGS, OTR/L, is an occupational therapist in private practice with clients with developmental delays. She is a retired Assistant Clinical Professor and Level I Fieldwork Supervisor at Boston University. She currently teaches as an adjunct instructor in the Occupational Therapy Assistant program at Bristol Community College. Her commitment to occupational therapy assistant/occupational therapist collaborative practices began through her work as the founder and past Program Chair of an occupational therapy assistant program. She has supervised occupational therapy assistant practitioners in her clinical experiences in both public schools and home health.

Cathie Marqusee, MS, OTR/L, is a practicing occupational therapist in public schools in Cambridge, Massachusetts. She has been an occupational therapist since 1987.

Kathryn Prizio, MS, OTR/L, has been an occupational therapist for 7 years, working with adult and geriatric patients in a variety of settings, including long-term acute care, skilled nursing facilities, and home heath. She is a graduate of Stonehill College, where she obtained her baccalaureate in psychology. She obtained her master's degree in occupational therapy from Boston School of Occupational Therapy at Tufts University in 2006. Special interests include working with complex medical patients and working with developmentally disabled inpatients.

Debra G. Sharp, MEd, is an educational specialist and consultant. She has a bachelor of science degree, with a focus on child development and an emphasis in communicative disorders, and a master of science degree in special education, with a focus on early childhood. She has worked in the education field for 20 years.

Kimberly Witkowski, MS, OTR/L, is an occupational therapist who works with adults in clinical settings. She attended the University of New Hampshire, graduating and entering the field of occupational therapy in 2009. She worked for 5 years for the Veterans Health Administration before taking a position in an outpatient clinic. Her primary clinical experience is in long-term care and outpatient services, including participation in the wheelchair clinic and falls committee.

PREFACE

This book was born out of our frustration as instructors that most case studies in current texts asked only for treatment plans and goals. The real-life situations that we saw as practicing therapists were not well represented in these case scenarios. Students were not asked to think about the steps after the treatment plan was completed and actual treatment had begun. This is, we feel, where a truly flexible and adaptable student does well on fieldwork, when he or she has the ability to realize that working with real clients requires flexibility, adaptability, and a sense of humor. Often, our best attempts to predict outcomes fail because of circumstances we did not anticipate during our initial evaluation—maybe because of family, health, or client-centered issues. Therefore, our goals for this textbook are to assist students in learning that there can be many possible choices in the clinical decision-making process and that these different choices can lead to many equally successful outcomes. Mental flexibility and thinking on one's feet are important clinical skills to cultivate, and students must learn that there are few black-and-white decisions in clinical practice. By developing these skills, one can cross the bridge between being a well-educated student and a competent clinical practitioner.

The second edition of this book has been revised to reflect the changes that have taken place since the first edition appeared. When the first edition was published, Uniform Terminology was what we used to understand the component skills for practice. This present edition is built around the *Occupational Therapy Practice Framework* (OTPF). It is purposely not identified with a specific *OTPF* because this document goes through periodic reviews, and we did not want to tie this edition to any specific edition of the *OTPF*. Using this framework, each case now asks students to consider the client's occupations, performance patterns, performance skills, client factors, contexts, and environments; the situations and discharge planning sections have remained. Additionally, we have included questions on theory and evidence. As the profession has moved toward theory-driven and evidenced-based practice, these questions will allow students to think of these concepts and search the literature to support their interventions.

Cases are also now formatted around an occupational profile and an analysis of occupation, again adhering to *OTPF* terminology. Each response to a question creates another clinical pathway for the student to examine; each response will affect the answer to the next question(s). The various pathways that develop allow students to compare their work and see that many responses can be appropriate for the same case.

The authors have included pediatric cases, more community cases, and one case in primary care, which is an emerging practice area. Although there is no case for an individual with autism, many of these are available in other textbooks. We made the decision to include conditions that are not found as commonly in pediatric textbooks.

This book is not intended to teach theories and constructs for clinical reasoning, nor is it meant to teach occupational therapy or occupational therapy assistant students how to evaluate. The students are expected to use the information provided by the occupational profile and analysis of occupation. Students should be able to explain the rationale for their answers to each question because this book is intended to provide a vehicle to put theories and clinical reasoning into practice before reaching the clinical fieldwork stage of training. Doing so will help students to reason out how to deal with the different scenarios they may encounter during their clinical placements. Although one can never be prepared for everything that may happen during fieldwork, we feel these cases offer a realistic picture of various clinical settings and raise the difficult questions that students may be asked.

We hope you find this edition to be a valuable learning tool for your students.

INTRODUCTION

We wrote this text as a workbook to encourage students' clinical reasoning skills. This book can be used in many ways and is only limited by the skill and imagination of the instructor. We purposely did not use a specific frame of reference or theoretical model in this book for several reasons. This allows each college or technical program to fit the book to its specific frames of reference or theoretical model and enables instructors to use various frames of reference and theories with different cases. In a few cases, assessments have been used that do pertain to a specific frame of reference or theory, including the Model of Human Occupation and the Allen Disability Levels. These questions can be easily rephrased with another frame of reference, or even deleted, if the instructor wishes to do so.

In many of the cases, we do not provide specific details. This is to encourage students to look up information and find resources outside of their classroom texts, which is a skill that they will need in clinical practice and as they further their clinical education. We encourage instructors to add or delete information to enhance or refocus a case or to adapt it to the academic level and knowledge base of their class. Instructors may have students complete cases or certain questions several times simply by adding or omitting details. This will allow them to compare the different clinical pathways, treatment, and outcomes when only one detail changes. Additionally, instructors may assign one half of the class a case with information deleted or changed and the other half with the information unchanged. This will generate interesting discussions, comparisons, and learning. We also encourage instructors to bring their own clinical experiences and theoretical orientation to the discussions of the cases.

For class use, cases can be assigned as group or individual projects, as work to be done during small discussion sections, or as assignments outside of class. In addition, the cases can be used to initiate discussions about different aspects of patient treatment. Although we have grouped the cases by settings, they do not need to be followed in this order.

We feel this textbook can be used in many different classes and even during the same semester by different classes. In examining input from various instructors, students can see how information is integrated from various course areas to provide holistic occupational therapy treatment. This is beneficial for the program because it enhances the curriculum and provides a connection between classes that is often missing. Cases may be completed several times by the same group of students as they progress through their coursework. This gives them the opportunity to compare how they would react to a situation as, for example, a first-year student and again as a second-year student. Allowing students to reflect on changes they might make with more knowledge and experience gives them the opportunity to grow as clinicians. Both professional and technical programs can use this text. For example, consider having classes in both a professional and a technical program work on the same case to explore how the registered occupational therapist–certified occupational therapist assistant relationship works.

Most important, students want to become competent therapists and are often hungry for the right answers. As instructors, we have all witnessed students who have gotten stuck when presented with information that does not have clear answers. As practicing therapists, we know the importance of realizing that occupational therapy is an evolving process. The therapeutic relationship and the occupational therapy intervention plan may change during this process. By understanding this, students can practice how to make the changes positive instead of trying to block them.

Again, students need to be reminded that there will be many answers to the same questions. They may find different answers among classmates and even among different instructors in the same program. They can then evaluate, with the help of their instructors, which responses they think will work best for the patient and for themselves as therapists. Doing so will also foster the development of the skills of therapeutic use of self.

We encourage instructors to be creative in the ways they use this workbook, to use it as a tool to encourage students to think "outside the box," and to help students understand that cookie-cutter treatments are not possible in occupational therapy.

I
Acute Care Hospital

Adam: Myocardial Infarction

OCCUPATIONAL PROFILE

Adam is a 56-year-old White man brought to the emergency department by his wife after complaining of chest pain, indigestion, and heartburn that had been going on for several hours. He was admitted to the coronary care unit (CCU) with a diagnosis of myocardial infarction (MI) and coronary artery disease. Before his MI, he was independent in all his daily life functions. He is a highly successful executive for a technology firm. He has been married for 31 years and has two sons; one son is away at college, and the second is a junior in high school. His wife, Janine, works full time as a chief financial officer for a chain of retail stores.

Adam and his family live in a large, two-story colonial home in the suburbs with four bedrooms and two full baths upstairs and a half bath and living areas on the first floor. He can enter the house from the garage up five steps. Once inside, he must manage a long flight of stairs to get to the second story.

Adam loves to golf and sail, and he takes his family on two vacations a year to exotic places to pursue these activities. He wakes early (around 5 a.m.) and comes home late

from work (around 9 p.m.). He drinks large amounts of coffee and smokes two packs of cigarettes a day. His father died at the age of 62 of a heart attack. Adam is a driven man who expects everyone around him to excel and to extend themselves to the fullest. He works an average of 70 hours a week. He enjoys his lifestyle and his roles as worker and father the most, although he spends little time with his family. He is a confident man and states that he does not let difficult situations get to him. Adam denies that stress is a factor in his life and says he thrives on challenges. He is planning to return home immediately after his hospitalization and to return to work quickly.

He is being seen by occupational therapy (OT) and physical therapy (PT) immediately after his discharge from the CCU onto the cardiac floor of the hospital.

ANALYSIS OF OCCUPATIONAL PERFORMANCE

Adam was evaluated 2 days after his MI. Evaluation included chart review, interview, and observation of

Lowenstein NA, Halloran P.
Case Studies Through the Health Care Continuum:
A Workbook for the Occupational Therapy Student, Second Edition (pp 3-5).
© 2015 SLACK Incorporated.

functional activity. His room is on the coronary care floor, not in the CCU. Adam's MI is of a moderate nature, with damage to the heart evident on electrocardiogram. Additional diagnoses include high cholesterol and tendonitis of the elbow. Adam has not had a physical in years and has no documented history of heart disease. Adam is 5'8" and weighs 200 pounds. He presents with no deficits in cognition, perception, sensation, vision, or hearing. He has active range of motion (ROM) within normal limits and good coordination; he is left-handed. His strength was not tested because of his cardiac status, but appears functional for current tasks. He has significant deficits in endurance, with his sitting tolerance out of bed only 5 minutes. He can transfer from the bed to the chair and from sit to stand with contact guard. Supine to sit requires supervision, and his bed mobility (rolling side to side) is independent using the bed rails to assist. He can ambulate without devices and walks short distances (bed to bathroom) before becoming short of breath.

Currently, Adam requires maximum assistance for dressing both his upper and lower body. He can wash his face and hands while sitting on the edge of his bed with setup of materials and a wash basin; he is contact guard for ambulation and independent for toilet hygiene. Instrumental activities of daily living (IADL) were not assessed at this time. He has been fearful and anxious since his MI. He feels he has lost control of his life. He does not want to die and has been thinking a lot of his father's early death from heart disease.

He is cooperative and wishes to actively participate in his rehab program and return home; he expects to be back at work within 2 weeks and says he does not trust the work to get done without him there. He has already started to contact the office by cell phone, and he has his laptop with him in his room. Adam's goals are to return home and to work as soon as possible. His expected length of stay is 1 week.

QUESTIONS

Occupations

1. Look at the *Occupational Therapy Practice Framework (OTPF)* and identify three to five areas of occupation that would be important to address either through client–family education or direct intervention. What leads you to believe these are important occupations to address before Adam is discharged home?

2. Prioritize the occupations you identified. Explain why your chose these. Did payment or setting factors influence your choices? How? Did you take into consideration Adam's choices?

3. Write a problem list for Adam indicating the issues that need to be addressed during his acute care hospital stay. Does this differ from the occupations you identified?

4. How would you address Adam's work role? What do you see as important issues for Adam to understand in this area?

5. How would you address Adam's leisure activities?

Performance Patterns

6. How do Adam's routines contribute to his health and well-being?

7. Would you recommend that Adam make any changes to his routines? If so, what recommendations would you make and why?

8. Adam's role as a worker is important to him. How would you educate him on the impact this role may have on his health?

Performance Skills

9. Identify five to eight performance skills that should be addressed during Adam's OT sessions.

10. Describe an intervention session to address three of your identified performance skills. What types of interventions are you using (e.g., occupation, activity or preparatory)?

11. Describe the patient education program for Adam concerning his activities of daily living (ADL) routine.

12. Given that Adam has a decrease in his endurance, what type of exercise program would you create to address this? Are you using preparatory methods and tasks, activity based tasks, or occupation based tasks?

Client Factors

13. What are the signs and symptoms of cardiac stress that you must watch for during your treatment sessions with Adam?

14. What vital signs should you monitor before, during, and after each treatment session, and how do you monitor them? What are the normal parameters for these vital signs?

15. Would you teach breathing techniques to use during his ADL routine? If so, what breathing techniques would you teach him, and how would you recommend that he incorporate these into his ADL routine?

16. What safety issues should you address with Adam regarding his return home?

17. Stress is an important risk factor in MI. How do you think OT should address this in treatment with Adam?

18. Identify any issues you feel affect Adam's psychological health. Why are these issues as important to address as his physical issues in his treatment?

19. Would you consider referring Adam to another discipline for psychosocial issues? If so, which one(s)?

Contexts and Environment

20. What, if any, adaptive equipment might you recommend for Adam to use during his ADL routine?

21. What would you recommend regarding Adam's work routine?

22. What type of adaptations would you recommend Adam make to his home? Would these adaptations be permanent or temporary?

23. What would you identify as important lifestyle changes, and how would you educate him in these areas?

Theory and Evidence

24. What theory/theories or frame(s) of reference might you use in developing an intervention plan? Describe the rationale for your choice(s).

25. What, if any, evidence can you find to support your choice of theory/theories or frame(s) of reference (or both)?

26. What, if any, evidence can you find to support intervention?

Intervention Plan and Goals

27. On the basis of the goals Adam has expressed, write a list of long- and short-term goals for OT intervention.

28. Do Adam's stated goals coincide with the OT goals? Why or why not?

29. What functional activities would you use to reach these goals?

30. Knowing that Adam's expected length of stay in the acute care hospital is only 1 week, what discharge plans would you recommend for Adam at this time?

31. Please write an intervention plan for Adam. Use the *OTPF* and include the intervention approaches and types.

Situations

32. Adam's wife asks to speak to you privately. She tells you that she is afraid to let Adam return to work, golf, or sailing and does not know how to get him to give up his leisure interests. How do you handle this situation?

33. Adam and his wife tell you they are afraid of resuming sexual activity. How do you handle this situation? How comfortable are you in dealing with this area and, if you are not comfortable, what course of action should you take?

34. You enter Adam's room to start treatment and find him on the phone with his office. He is agitated and angry. When he gets off the phone, you take his blood pressure and find that it is 200/120. How do you handle this situation?

35. Adam tells you that he wants to start a daily exercise routine and purchase some equipment for his home. What do you suggest he purchase, if anything?

36. You recommend that Adam return to the hospital as an outpatient and participate in the stress management classes and cardiac rehab program that are offered. He says that he thrives on the intensity and does not find it stressful. How do you respond to this?

Discharge Planning

37. How would you address Adam's insistence that he return to work after his hospital stay and not go to the hospital's cardiac rehab program?

38. Given that Adam insists on going home and returning to work instead of attending a cardiac rehab program, what would your discharge instructions include?

Craig: Spinal Cord Injury, C-5

OCCUPATIONAL PROFILE

Craig is a 36-year-old Asian man who fell off a ladder while fixing a sign at the retail cell phone store he owns. His employee saw the fall and called 911 after it was clear that Craig could not get up. He was transported to the nearest emergency department, where he had a magnetic resonance imaging (MRI) scan that indicated that he had sustained a complete fracture of the spinal cord at the C-5 level. Craig is in good health and has no other known medical conditions. He was placed in the intensive care unit (ICU) to await surgery for a halo vest. After 2 days, it was felt that Craig was medically stable, and surgery was performed to place him in the halo vest. He was transferred out of the ICU onto a medical unit.

Craig is married and has no children; he and his wife were waiting until Craig's store was financially stable before starting a family. Craig opened his cell phone store 18 months ago, which sells phones, plans, and accessories, and provides customer support. Craig has two part-time employees, and he spends about 70 hours a week at the store, working at least 6 days a week. His wife, Elaine, works full time as a receptionist in a doctor's office. They live in a

large city in a fifth-floor apartment; there is an elevator in the building. Their apartment is a small one-bedroom, with one bathroom and a galley kitchen; the living room doubles as a dining area.

Craig's and Elaine's families live in nearby communities. Their families are immigrants from Korea; both Craig and Elaine are first-generation Americans and speak English well, but their families are more comfortable with Korean as their main language, especially when in crisis. Their families are proud of them and their achievements. Both families are devastated by the news of Craig's accident. Family ties are close, and Craig's parents continue to hold beliefs from their Korean culture about family and health. Craig has two sisters. One lives nearby and works full time, and the other is currently living and working in Korea.

Craig is a quiet, confident man. He is soft-spoken with a wry sense of humor. He has an optimistic outlook on his life. Craig believes that hard work and persistence will lead to success. He is a college graduate. He and his wife have a strong marriage and share the same cultural heritage and beliefs. He is bilingual, speaking both English and Korean fluently. His leisure interests include biking and hiking. Craig worked in retail before starting his own business. He hopes his business will be able to support his family so that

Lowenstein NA, Halloran P.
Case Studies Through the Health Care Continuum:
A Workbook for the Occupational Therapy Student, Second Edition (pp 7-10).
© 2015 SLACK Incorporated.

his wife can stop working when they have children. Craig's goals are to return to his business and home.

ANALYSIS OF OCCUPATIONAL PERFORMANCE

Craig was seen by OT immediately after the halo vest was applied. Evaluation included observation, sensation testing, and motor testing. No formal cognitive or perceptual assessments were performed; however, he demonstrates no deficits in cognition, perception, vision, or hearing on observation and interviews. His sensation is absent distal to C-5. In addition, he is dependent for all ADL, transfers, and mobility. Craig has flaccid paralysis throughout his upper extremities (UEs) and lower extremities (LEs).

Craig had been immobilized on a kinetic bed until his halo vest was applied; he was able to tolerate supported sitting up for 10 minutes during the evaluation, before he began to complain of feeling nauseous and dizzy. Craig asked to continue the evaluation at another time. During the OT evaluation, he appeared despondent, angry, and confused. He does not seem to understand what a complete spinal cord injury means and is frustrated that no one will tell him if he will walk or hug his wife again. His goal for therapy is to do what he must to get to the rehabilitation hospital. His expected length of stay is 2 weeks if no medical complications arise. He is being seen by OT and PT. His insurance is workers' compensation.

QUESTIONS

Occupations

1. What areas of occupation would you address during Craig's acute care stay? Why?

2. Given Craig's current emotional state, what occupation might you introduce to give Craig and his wife hope for the future?

3. What might you address in the area of self-care with Craig during his 2-week stay? Why did you choose this area?

4. Given the level of Craig's injury, do you think he will eventually be able to dress himself? Explain your answer.

5. Given Craig's business, do you think he can successfully return to his store after rehabilitation? Give the rationale for your answer.

Performance Patterns

6. How would you educate yourself about cultural factors that may be important for Craig's recovery and your intervention planning?

7. How have Craig's roles been affected by his accident? What can you do to help him with one of these roles while in the acute care hospital?

Performance Skills

8. Identify 8 to 10 performance skills that should be addressed during Craig's OT sessions.

9. Given the level of Craig's injury, what motor skills might he be able to perform? What functional tasks could these motor skills influence? How?

10. Describe an intervention session to address three of your identified performance skills. What types of interventions are you using (e.g., occupation, activity, preparatory)?

11. How might you address Craig's emotional state?

Client Factors

12. Given the level of Craig's injury, which muscles would be fully innervated, and which muscles would be partially innervated? What motions would Craig have in his UEs?

13. How would you assess Craig's upper UE status?

14. What is the name of the severe medical emergency that can be life-threatening to a spinal cord injury patient? What are its symptoms, and what are the actions you should take if this happens when you are working with Craig?

15. What is orthostatic hypotension? What are its symptoms, and what should you do if Craig experiences this while you are working with him? What precautions must be taken with Craig, given his immobilization in bed?

16. How will you instruct Craig in pressure relief? Why is it important for Craig to learn to do this? What other discipline would be responsible for education in this area?

17. Why does Craig have flaccid paralysis? Is this common in spinal cord injury? Will spasticity develop in his muscles?

18. What interventions would you do with Craig to address his flaccid paralysis?

19. What type of splint would you make for Craig, and what is the goal of wearing the splint? Write out a wearing schedule for Craig's splint. What should staff be educated to look for when taking off his splint?

20. How will OT assist Craig in developing sitting tolerance? Explain your treatment techniques.

21. What is the safest method to use in transferring Craig from his bed to his wheelchair?

22. What treatments might OT and PT work on together? How can you document this to be sure there is no duplication of service?

23. Discuss the stages of psychological adjustment to physical disabilities. What stage do you feel Craig is experiencing?

24. What are some of the common coping mechanisms that individuals use in dealing with traumatic injury? Comment on the positive or negative impact each may have on recovery.

25. What psychosocial supports are currently available to help Craig deal with his emotional state?

Contexts and Environment

26. Given that Craig's parents are traditional Koreans, what might some of their health beliefs entail? How would you go about ascertaining how Craig's, his wife's, and his parent's cultural beliefs might influence intervention?

27. What are important aspects of Craig's personal and temporal contexts to consider?

28. What, if any, adaptive equipment might you give Craig in the acute care hospital? Why?

29. Write a prescription for or identify a wheelchair for Craig. This should include the type of wheelchair, any customized seating systems, controls, or other features.

30. What are your considerations regarding Craig's mobility in relation to his current living situation? His business?

31. Would you recommend any assistive technology for Craig at this time? Why or why not?

32. The acute care hospital is the first environment where Craig, his wife, and their families will learn about spinal cord injury. What types of information would you give them at this time? Where will you look for information? Can you find any organizations or support groups in your area for spinal cord injuries? Write them here.

33. There are several risks associated with spinal cord injury, and Craig and his wife need to do daily checks for some of these. What are these risks, and how do you educate Craig and his wife about them?

34. Craig's wife wants to be an integral part of his care. What activities can she do for him to help maintain his musculoskeletal integrity?

Theory and Evidence

35. What theory/theories or frame(s) of reference might you use in developing an intervention plan? Describe the rationale for your choice(s).

36. What, if any, evidence can you find to support your choice of theory/theories and/or frame(s) of reference?

37. What, if any, evidence can you find to support intervention?

Intervention Plan and Goals

38. Given that you were unable to complete the OT evaluation, what additional information would be needed to devise an intervention plan?

39. Write a problem list for Craig. How would you prioritize these problems? Did you take into account Craig's or his family's wishes?

40. Write a list of three long-term goals.

41. Write a list of four short-terms goals to align with each long-term goal.

Situations

42. You are working with Craig and he starts to perspire, complaining of a pounding headache and chills. What does this indicate, and what is your response?

43. During treatment sessions, Craig talks constantly about the day that he will walk. It motivates him to participate in his OT sessions and gives him hope. How might you handle this?

44. Craig has developed moderate spasticity in his LEs and mild spasticity in his UEs. He is anxious about this change and thinks this means he is getting worse. How might you explain the presence of spasticity to him? How can spasticity be useful in your treatment program?

45. One afternoon, you enter Craig's room to find it filled with family members from both sides. They have set up a small shrine and seem to be involved in some sort of religious practice. Your schedule is tight, and this is the only time you have to see Craig in the afternoon. What do you do?

Discharge Planning

46. Craig has been at the acute care hospital for 2 weeks and is ready for discharge to a rehabilitation facility. Write a discharge summary using the following information: Craig is currently in a hospital-owned power chair 2 hours a day; his power chair has been ordered. He has had several episodes of orthostatic hypotension and autonomic dysreflexia and has developed spasticity. Include other information from the case history and contexts.

Paul: Total Knee Replacement

OCCUPATIONAL PROFILE

Paul is an 89-year-old man who lives in a large city with his 87-year-old wife of 65 years. He was admitted to the acute care hospital for voluntary knee replacement surgery of his right knee. Paul and his wife have three adult children, one who lives in the same city, and two who live out of town, each about 4 hours away. His children are all supportive and involved with both their parents' care. Paul and his wife have six grandchildren, scattered around the country. Paul has been retired from his job as a fundraiser for a nonprofit agency for more than 15 years. He is the primary caretaker in the family because his wife has severe depression and short-term memory loss. They have a companion who works 3 days a week for 3 to 4 hours each day to assist with Paul's wife's hygiene and with meal preparation. Paul is independent in his ADLs and has assistance with hot meal preparation, although he enjoys making light meals from the food he buys at the neighborhood markets. He enjoys going out in his neighborhood and shopping at gourmet food stores and grocery shopping; however, his mobility has become more limited because of his deterio-

rating right knee. He likes to watch sports and the news on television, and to read the daily newspapers. Paul used to enjoy concerts and shows and going to lectures, but he gave these up because his wife would call his cell phone every 10 minutes wondering where he was and when he was coming home. They live in a large (2,000 square feet) apartment (all on one floor). There are three bedrooms and two and a half bathrooms. There are no grab bars; the bathtubs double as showers and have sliding glass doors. The toilets have a toilet frame for holding onto when getting on and off the toilet. The apartment building has three steps to get into the building with handrails on one side and then an elevator to get to the apartment. There is a 24-hour doorman who will help with bags and other items as needed. Because Paul and his wife have lived in the building for more than 50 years, the members of the building staff are eager to assist him. His goal is to return home and resume taking care of his wife and to go shopping in the neighborhood. He is being seen by PT and OT in the acute care hospital. Paul has Medicare Part A and Part B for his insurance and wants to return home to continue his rehabilitation.

Lowenstein NA, Halloran P.
Case Studies Through the Health Care Continuum:
A Workbook for the Occupational Therapy Student, Second Edition (pp 11-13).
© 2015 SLACK Incorporated.

ANALYSIS OF OCCUPATIONAL PERFORMANCE

On day 1 post-surgery, an OT evaluation was completed, based on functional activity and observation. Paul was able to wash his upper body while sitting in bed with setup on a bedside table. He required moderate assistance to move to the edge of the bed and dangle his legs. Transfer between bed and chair required a maximum assist of 2 with non–weight-bearing on his right leg using a walker. Paul is alert and oriented, although at night he has had some delusions that he is in the middle of an earthquake and that he is at a banquet in some hall. For safety, he has an aide with him 24 hours a day while he is having the delusions at night. Paul's wife visits daily and stays for 8 hours, sitting in a chair in his room. The companion accompanies her to the hospital and also sits in the room. Daily PT is working on transfers from bed to stand and ambulation with a walker. His length of stay is expected to be 1 week.

QUESTIONS

Occupations

1. What occupations can you focus on given the short time frame that you have with Paul in acute care? Why are these important to address before his discharge?

2. What priority order would you put them in and why?

3. Write a problem list for Paul of the issues that need to be addressed during his acute care hospital stay.

Performance Patterns

4. Paul's role as caregiver is important to him. What immediate impact does his knee replacement have on this role?

5. Given Paul's age, what are your expectations for his ability to return to his previous level of function? Explain your reasoning.

Performance Skills

6. Identify five to eight performance skills that should be addressed during Paul's OT sessions.

7. Describe an intervention session to address three of your identified performance skills. What types of interventions would you use (e.g., occupation, activity, or preparatory)?

Client Factors

8. Identify 10 key body functions that are affected by Paul's knee replacement.

9. Do you feel Paul requires exercises for his UEs while in the acute care hospital? Why? If so, which exercises would you teach him?

10. Would you monitor Paul's vital signs during your OT intervention sessions? Why or why not?

Contexts and Environment

11. What precautions would you need to adhere to during your OT sessions? How would you teach Paul about these precautions?

12. Are there any safety issues you should address regarding his return home? Who would you talk to about these?

13. What, if any, adaptive equipment might you recommend for Paul to use during his ADL routine?

14. What type of adaptations would you recommend that Paul make to his home? Would these adaptations be permanent or temporary?

15. What type of patient education would you provide for Paul? Would you also provide this education to anyone else? Who?

Theory and Evidence

16. What theory/theories or frame(s) of reference might you use in developing an intervention plan? Describe the rationale for your choice(s).

17. What, if any, evidence can you find to support your choice of theory/theories and/or frame(s) of reference?

18. What, if any, evidence can you find to support intervention?

Intervention Plan and Goals

19. Write a problem list for Paul, noting the issues that need to be addressed during his acute care hospital stay.

20. Write three long-term and short-term goals for OT intervention.

21. Write an intervention plan for Paul. Use the *OTPF* and include the intervention methods and activities.

Situations

22. You enter Paul's room and find him slowly moving his arms in front of his face. When you ask him what is he doing, he tells you that he is trying to remove the spider web from the room. What medical issue(s) might be the cause of his hallucination?

23. Paul's wife is sitting in his room, and you start to transfer him from his bed to a chair so he can begin a sponge bath of his upper body. His wife tells you that he does not need to know how to do that because she will take care of him. However, you are aware that she does not do any caretaking. You have never been in Paul's room without his wife being there. How would you handle this situation?

Discharge Planning

24. Where would you recommend Paul go for discharge? Why?

25. Paul insists that he only wants to go home for his rehabilitation. You believe he will need extensive assistance and do not support this, but his family is insistent. What would you recommend to ensure his safety?

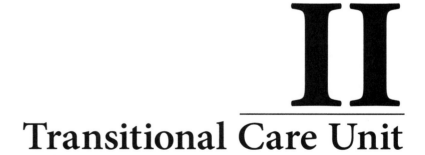

II
Transitional Care Unit

4

Kim: Coronary Artery Bypass Graft and Congestive Heart Failure

OCCUPATIONAL PROFILE

Kim is a 63-year-old, divorced Black woman. She underwent a coronary artery bypass graft (CABG) involving three arteries 2 weeks ago. Kim had been experiencing chest pain with minimal exertion and was diagnosed with three blocked coronary arteries. She underwent the CABG procedure at a large teaching hospital. She has additional diagnoses of congestive heart failure, diabetes, hypothyroidism, and schizophrenia.

Kim lives in a second floor walk-up apartment with her parrot, Cleo, and her dog, Casey. She works part time as a clerk in a convenience store, and her responsibilities include moving boxes, stocking the shelves, and managing the cash register. Kim received a diagnosis of schizophrenia when she was a sophomore in college and was never able to complete her degree. Both of her parents are deceased and she has one sister who lives far away, but with whom she has a good relationship. She attends a day hospital program 2 days a week where she has a case manager and a psychologist. She takes medication for her schizophrenia and does well as long as she does not stop taking it. She drives short distances for errands, such as grocery shopping and doing her laundry (there are no laundry facilities in the apartment building). She is a private person and does not know anyone in her building.

Kim has been independent in all of her life tasks; however, a few months before her surgery, she started to tire easily and was not able to do as much as usual. Kim has few friends. She does not go out much socially and has a limited support system. She is a quiet person and has difficulty making friends as she does not feel comfortable in social situations. Kim loves animals, and her pets are like her family. She dotes on both animals—buying them special treats and taking Casey on walks as Cleo rides on Kim's shoulder. She worries about her animals while she is on the transitional care unit. She is planning on returning home to her pets and hopes to return to work and to the day program. She is being seen by OT, PT, and daily nursing care. Her recovery in acute care has been unremarkable from a medical perspective, and she was transferred to a transitional care unit for further rehabilitation. Her length of stay is expected to be 2 weeks. She receives Medicaid.

Lowenstein NA, Halloran P.
Case Studies Through the Health Care Continuum:
A Workbook for the Occupational Therapy Student, Second Edition (pp 17-20).
© 2015 SLACK Incorporated.

ANALYSIS OF OCCUPATIONAL PERFORMANCE

Kim was evaluated by the occupational therapist on the day of admission and the following morning through observation, interview, chart review, and manual muscle testing. No formal cognitive or perceptual testing was completed. Kim wears bifocal glasses. Her hearing, sensation, and perception all appear intact by observation, but formal assessment was not conducted. She appears to be forgetful about recent information. Her active ROM in both UEs is within normal limits. Her strength is 3+ of 5 throughout both UEs. She has no deficits in coordination and is right-handed. Her endurance is poor for all functional activities. She continues to have pain (6 on a scale of 1 to 10) in the sternum. She fatigues easily and only tolerates 15 minutes out of bed at a time. She has pain from the incision on her chest. Her skin is intact except for on the surgical site, which is healing well.

Kim can roll in bed using the bedrails and can only move from sit to supine by first raising the head of the bed. She transfers from sit to stand with the moderate assist of one, and ambulates using a rolling walker because of LE weakness. Kim has refused to dress in anything more than a hospital gown. She will wash her hands and face sitting up in bed, but then is too tired to continue and allows the staff to complete her bathing. She is eating little and she claims she does not have much appetite. She is worried about her pets and asks if she can have them brought to the hospital at every intervention session. Her case manager is taking care of them while she is hospitalized.

She has expressed to all staff members that her goals are to return home to her animals. She is willing to participate in intervention, but just "doesn't have the energy."

QUESTIONS

Occupations

1. Make a list of the key occupations that Kim wants to work on. Make a list of the key occupations that you feel she should work on. What are the similarities and differences in the two lists?

2. What types of equipment and facilities would it be helpful for the hospital to have to work on some of these occupations?

3. Are there any concerns regarding Kim's ability to drive after her return home? What other types of transportation might be available to Kim if she is unable to drive?

Performance Patterns

4. What routines do you feel have been most affected by Kim's cardiac condition and why?

5. How can OT assist Kim in these areas?

6. What roles have been affected by Kim's cardiac condition? Describe how OT might assist Kim in resuming or adapting these roles.

7. How would you recommend that Kim adapt her daily morning routine to compensate for her poor endurance?

8. What techniques should Kim be taught to help her manage her energy during her recovery?

Performance Skills

9. Identify five motor, process, and social interaction performance skills that are important to address during Kim's rehabilitation. Why did you identify these in particular?

10. How would you address Kim's bathing skills? Describe how you would grade the activity and progress from her current level to being able to bathe seated at the sink.

11. Because Kim is planning to return home, what type of kitchen activity would you plan for your first session in the kitchen? Why? What performance skills are important for you to assess and address for this activity?

12. What part of the dressing task do you think would be most difficult for Kim to accomplish and why? Do you think Kim's surgery will affect her ability to perform this job? If so, how?

13. Write out an exercise program using activity and occupation intervention methods to improve Kim's UE strength. How would you document this so it pertains to OT?

14. Describe two intervention activities that you could do to increase Kim's endurance (at least one of these needs to be an activity or occupation intervention method). Why did you choose them? Did you consider Kim's interests when planning them?

15. Kim is having difficulty remembering to use energy conservation and breathing techniques during her morning routine. What techniques could you use to address this issue?

Client Factors

16. What are some psychosocial issues for Kim? How would you incorporate working on these into your intervention sessions?

17. Given what you know about Kim's psychological status, how well do you think she is coping with her current condition? What would you do to assist her in this area?

18. What concerns do you have in relation to Kim's diagnosis of schizophrenia?

19. How would you address Kim's bed mobility issues? Why is it important to address this mobility challenge early in intervention?

20. For what reasons should Kim's blood pressure and pulse be monitored during therapy?

21. At what blood pressure reading would you stop activity? How long would you wait to see if her blood pressure came down? What would you do in regard to notifying other team members of a high blood pressure reading?

22. Other than pulse and blood pressure, what are some other concerns to be aware of?

Contexts and Environment

23. Would you recommend any adaptive equipment for Kim to take home? If so, what and why?

24. Your supervisor has asked you to help develop an educational group for patients who have undergone CABG. Each discipline (OT, nursing, PT, social work, nutrition) will lead a 1-hour session. What would you do for the OT session and why?

25. What type of patient education material would you give to Kim and why?

26. Identify two websites that would be of benefit to Kim. Why did you choose these?

27. What physical and social supports might you find for Kim?

28. Identify personal and temporal factors to take into consideration during Kim's OT intervention. Why did you identify these as important?

Theory and Evidence

29. What theory/theories or frame(s) of reference might you use in developing an intervention plan? Describe the rationale for your choices.

30. What, if any, evidence can you find to support your choice of theory/theories and/or frame(s) of reference?

31. What, if any, evidence can you find to support intervention?

Intervention Plan and Goals

32. Using the Model of Human Occupation, how would you assess Kim's volition and habituation?

33. Make a problem list for Kim, and put the problems in priority according to her goals.

34. Write the long- and short-term goals for the first three problems on your problem list.

35. What types of OT interventions will you plan to achieve your short-term goals? Would you use occupation, activities, or preparatory methods and tasks?

36. Could you take one of your preparatory intervention methods and achieve the same outcome with an activity or occupation method or task? Describe the new intervention.

37. What part of the intervention planning process could a certified occupational therapist assistant (COTA) participate in? What aspects of this intervention plan could a COTA carry out?

38. Should you administer a standardized cognitive assessment and, if so, which one? What type of cognitive issues might you expect and why?

Situations

39. Kim has consistently expressed a desire to go home and to return to work, but is just as consistently not making progress in therapy. She continues to complain of fatigue and feeling too tired to participate. How would you deal with this issue, and with which other team members might you confer?

40. Kim has no clothing at the transitional care unit, and you would like to start working on dressing skills. She does not want to ask anyone to bring in clothes, even though her case manager has a key to her apartment. How would you address this issue?

41. You are in the middle of working on showering with Kim one morning. She starts to complain of chest pain and shortness of breath. She stops washing, catches her breath, and resumes the activity. After a few minutes, she again gets short of breath, but does not complain of chest pain. What should you do?

42. Kim keeps forgetting to pace herself during her ADL routine. Every time you work with her, you must remind her that she has to slow down. If she continues at the pace she sets, she gets short of breath and has to rest. How do you handle this situation?

43. During an exercise group, you notice that Kim is making comments as though she is talking to someone else in the room. She seems distracted and unable to focus on the exercise. You ask her whom she is talking to, and she tells you she is talking to her mother. What would you do?

Discharge Planning

44. Kim has progressed enough that she is able to return home. She is now able to wash at the sink while seated and can tolerate being out of bed for up to 4 hours. She has improved UE muscle strength to 4/5. She can make a light meal (toast, coffee, sandwich) using energy-conservation techniques. She can put on a hospital gown, but still has not attempted to get fully dressed because she has had no clothing with her. Write a referral for continued OT in home care.

45. On the basis of the description of Kim's status at discharge (see Question 44), which of the initial long-term goals that you set have been achieved? What might have been reasons that your other goals were not met?

5

Lyle: Right Total Knee Replacement

Occupational Profile

Lyle is a 57-year-old Black man with a diagnosis of a right total knee replacement. Lyle has a past medical history that includes morbid obesity, coronary artery disease, and hypertension. Lyle had elective knee replacement surgery because of pain in the right knee and decreased mobility.

Before the surgery, Lyle was independent with all self-care using several adaptive devices, including a reacher, a long-handled shoehorn, and a handheld shower head. He was independent in home management and community mobility skills. He ambulated with a limp, but used no device. Lyle works full time as an account representative for a corporation that manufactures institutional kitchen equipment. Lyle's job requires much travel, and he spends most of his time in the car and on the telephone. He reports that his job takes most of his time and that he works close to 60 hours per week, including all his travel time. With his company's recent downsizing, he now covers an even larger geographic area, but he "dares not complain" for fear of losing his job. He says he only has a few more years until retirement and plans to keep working until then. Lyle is concerned about the amount of time he has to lose from work because of the surgery and hopes to get back as soon as he is able. He says, laughing nervously, "I don't want to give them a chance to realize they'd be better off without me."

Lyle is divorced with three grown children. His youngest daughter, Chloe, moved in with him recently after her own divorce. She works full time and attends college part time in the evenings. Lyle lives in a two-story condominium where the bedrooms and bathroom are on the second floor. Lyle says he wants to move somewhere that has everything on one floor, but the condominium is so convenient to his office and he does not want to drive any more during the day than he has to.

Lyle is a large man, standing 5'10" tall and weighing close to 300 pounds. His lifestyle is hectic, and he admits to doing little to take care of himself. He claims he has no time for exercising or eating right. His physician has been trying to get him to lose weight for a while, with little luck. Although he has always been overweight, Lyle has been putting on weight recently. He feels this is due to more time spent in the car, his sedentary lifestyle, stress related to his

Lowenstein NA, Halloran P.
Case Studies Through the Health Care Continuum:
A Workbook for the Occupational Therapy Student, Second Edition (pp 21-24).
© 2015 SLACK Incorporated.

work, and his recent divorce from his wife of 31 years. He says he realizes the excess weight is what has expedited the deterioration of the right knee. His plan is to return to his current living situation and to work as soon as he is capable of doing so.

ANALYSIS OF OCCUPATIONAL PERFORMANCE

OT evaluation was completed by chart review, interview, and observation. Upon evaluation, Lyle is cooperative and talkative. He presents with no cognitive, perceptual, sensory, visual, or hearing deficits. He has functional use of both UEs; however, the ROM in his shoulders is limited slightly by his large body mass. He has no coordination or strength deficits and is right-hand dominant.

Lyle has a great deal of pain in the right knee. He gets relief from pain medication and takes the maximum dosage allowed daily. He complains of a dull pain when he is not moving and of excruciating pain in the right knee during all right UE motion. His knee is edematous and red, and the incision is covered with a dressing that nursing changes twice a day. Lyle is being watched closely for any signs of infection or deep vein thrombosis.

The mobility portion of the OT evaluation is completed with the physical therapist in case two people are needed to assist. Lyle is able to roll independently in the bed with the use of the bed rails. He requires minimum assistance to sit up from supine. He wears a knee immobilizer on the right leg to stabilize it during transfers. He is allowed touch-down weight bearing on the right leg and is to wear the knee immobilizer at all times except during exercises and while using the continuous passive motion machine. Lyle transfers from bed to chair with moderate assistance and performs commode transfers with the maximum assist of one, needing help with managing his clothing. Lyle uses a standard walker for all transfers. At this time, he is not walking, and is only performing stand-pivot transfers from one place to another. He fatigues quickly after transfers. Shower transfers are not attempted during the evaluation. Lyle uses a manual wheelchair and can propel it independently.

Lyle is able to feed and groom himself, as well as dress and bathe his upper body independently. He requires maximum assistance for all lower body care. He cannot reach his right foot while wearing the knee immobilizer and admits that this was hard for him to do even before the surgery. He is unable to perform any kitchen or home management tasks at the time of the evaluation.

Lyle is eager to begin therapy and agrees to participate in "whatever I need to do to go home." Lyle states that his goals for OT are to shower and dress himself and be able to make coffee. His only stipulation to participation is that the therapist coordinate with the nurse to be sure he has his pain medication before he is expected to do any kind of therapy. "I'd like to have as little pain as possible!" he remarks. It is anticipated that he will be at the unit for rehabilitation for 1 to 1.5 weeks. Upon discharge, he will continue with outpatient PT. Lyle has a private insurance plan that allows for 2 weeks of inpatient therapy.

QUESTIONS

Occupation

1. Look at the *OTPF* and identify three to five areas of occupation that would be important to address either through client/family education or direct intervention. What leads you to believe these are important occupations to address before Lyle is discharged home?

2. Prioritize the occupations you identified in Question 1. Explain why you chose these. Did payment or setting factors influence your choices? How? Did you take into consideration Lyle's choices?

3. How would you help Lyle make progress in his ability to bathe and dress before going home?

4. What portion of the ADL tasks do you anticipate will be most difficult for Lyle to accomplish?

5. How would you address Lyle's work role? What do you see as important issues for Lyle to understand in this area?

6. How would you design a session with Lyle to prepare a light snack using the microwave? What part of the snack preparation do you anticipate would be the most difficult for Lyle? Why?

Performance Patterns

7. Identify key roles that have been disrupted by Lyle's knee replacement.

8. What routines have been disrupted or are still intact?

9. What adaptations to his lifestyle might Lyle have to make to return to work?

10. In what ways could OT assist Lyle in fitting exercise into his daily routine?

Performance Skills

11. Identify five to eight performance skills that should be addressed during Lyle's OT sessions.

12. Describe an intervention session to address three of your identified performance skills. What types of interventions are you using (e.g., occupation, activity, or preparatory)?

Client Factors

13. Identify five client factors that are priorities for Lyle's OT intervention.

14. What concerns do you think Lyle has regarding his temporary functional limitations?

15. What are some ways to support Lyle psychologically to help him deal with his decreased mobility and function?

16. What type of instruction does Lyle need to promote recovery?

17. What are the precautions for a total knee replacement?

Contexts and Environment

18. Which of Lyle's values and beliefs is it important to consider during OT interventions?

19. What are some safety issues that might arise for Lyle?

20. How could you work with Lyle and the other team members to reduce the safety risk?

21. What type of adaptive equipment would Lyle need to maximize his independence?

22. Given that his estimated length of stay is 1 to 1.5 weeks, what equipment might Lyle need at home to maximize independence?

23. Explain how you would go about ordering such equipment for Lyle, keeping in mind his insurer. How would you find out what his insurance company would cover for durable medical equipment?

24. How might you involve Lyle's family to help him meet his goals?

25. Given what you know about Lyle's living situation, what adaptations might need to be made at his home for him to function?

26. What questions could you ask to determine whether Lyle might need adaptation equipment at work?

27. Would you want to look at Lyle's car? Why?

28. How might you adapt this portion of the ADL routine to maximize independence?

29. Lyle reports feeling bored on the unit because he is not used to "doing nothing." How would you address his leisure needs?

Theory and Evidence

30. What theory/theories or frame(s) of reference might you use in developing an intervention plan? Describe the rationale for your choices.

31. What, if any, evidence can you find to support your choice of theory/theories and/or frame(s) of reference?

32. What, if any, evidence can you find to support intervention?

Intervention Plan and Goals

33. Write out a problem list for Lyle.

34. Write out a list of Lyle's strengths.

35. What goals would you and Lyle set for his OT intervention?

36. What difficulties might you anticipate in Lyle meeting his goals?

37. How might you collaborate with other team members to incorporate OT goals into Lyle's program at the transitional care unit?

38. Write out a specific intervention plan for Lyle, including frequency.

Situations

39. You enter Lyle's room and find him trying to get to the bathroom by himself without the knee immobilizer on. What might you say to him, and what would you do?

40. Lyle tells you he was trying to get to the bathroom alone because two nursing assistants had come in and told him to wait a minute, and he had been waiting for almost 40 minutes. How would you respond to his comment?

41. Would you address his statement with any other staff members? Why? If you did decide to address it with someone, who would it be?

42. You enter Lyle's room at 8:30 a.m. to begin an ADL intervention. Lyle tells you he still has not had his 7:00 a.m. pain medication and cannot start until at least 30 minutes after he's had it. You have a busy morning with other ADL interventions and cannot reschedule him for later. What do you do?

43. You again set a time to see Lyle and his pain medication is not given to him before therapy as it is supposed to be. Lyle refuses therapy again and is angry about the situation. What would you do?

44. Lyle has been on pain medication for several months (he started taking it before his surgery). He refuses to participate in any therapies without having taken his pain medications at least 30 minutes to 1 hour before his therapy. At this point in his recovery, you have noted that he is still dependent on his pain medication. How would you approach this topic and with whom?

Discharge Planning

45. When would you begin discharge planning with Lyle?

46. What would you need to review with Lyle's daughter, Chloe, before he returns home?

47. What would you do if Lyle decided 2 days before the planned discharge date that he was leaving to go home? What factors may have led him to make that decision?

48. If you felt Lyle was not ready to leave, what course of action might you take? What would you say to Lyle?

49. At what level of function would you feel Lyle would need to be in order to be discharged home safely?

50. Would you recommend continued OT services for Lyle after discharge? Explain why or why not.

51. Write out a home program for Lyle.

Mary: Left Total Hip Replacement, Osteoarthritis

OCCUPATIONAL PROFILE

Mary is a 72-year-old White woman of Italian descent who recently underwent a left hip replacement. She also has osteoarthritis, hypertension, and a history of urinary tract infections. Mary had elective replacement surgery at the urging of her orthopedic surgeon because she had been suffering with progressively worse pain in the left hip over the past 2 years and had finally decided she could not tolerate it any longer. She had canceled the surgery once before, thinking she could do without it.

Mary has been becoming noticeably less active because of the hip pain for the past 8 months. Before hospitalization, Mary had been independent in all her meaningful occupations; however, she did mention that it has been taking her much longer to do her morning routine and daily tasks because of the hip pain. She had been able to ambulate without a device until approximately 2 months ago, when she decided to borrow a cane from her sister and use it "to lean on." She also found herself going upstairs only when she had to, such as to use the bathroom. Mary admits to cutting down on her coffee in the morning and other drinks throughout the day to help keep the trips to the

bathroom to a minimum. She also has reduced her errand running and driving and has been sleeping poorly because of anxiety over the surgery and the outcome. Mary is a religious woman and has attended the same church for more than 35 years. Mary lives alone in the suburbs in her own home, which has 5 stairs in the entrance and 12 stairs to the second floor where her bedroom and the only bathroom are; the laundry room is in the basement, which has a steep wooden staircase with only one handrail, on the left side. She has never been married and has no children. Mary has a sister who lives within walking distance from her home, but Mary says she started driving over recently instead of walking the two blocks for the visit.

Mary moved to the United States from Italy 55 years ago. She had been a nanny and a preschool teacher most of her career and retired 7 years ago at age 65. She had been socially active before her surgery. She plays cribbage once a week with three other women and is a volunteer at the town library, where she conducts children's reading and story hours. She is distressed that the story times are going to be canceled because of her surgery and spoke with hostility of the others at the library for not filling in while she is in the hospital. Mary is a kind woman with a strong sense of right and wrong. She speaks frequently about how wrong it

Lowenstein NA, Halloran P.
Case Studies Through the Health Care Continuum:
A Workbook for the Occupational Therapy Student, Second Edition (pp 25-28).
© 2015 SLACK Incorporated.

is to allow the children to go without their stories and how wrong it is for the others at the library to be so selfish. Mary seems to have a hard time letting go of feelings that bother her, and she deals with it by talking about it with anyone who will listen. She can often be seen telling the housekeepers and dietary aides as they enter and exit her room about the inconsideration of the other library volunteers. Mary seems to use her issue of choice to avoid conversations regarding her surgery and recovery.

Mary had an uncomplicated total hip replacement surgery. The acetabulum and femoral head and neck were replaced using a posterolateral approach. Mary has had no complications from her surgery and was moved from the acute portion of the hospital to the transitional care unit after 3 days. Mary initially hoped she would be able to go home directly after surgery. She agreed to move onto the transitional care unit after she and her sister realized that she would not be able to be at home safely. Mary's goals for her stay are to return home, to be able to drive, and to resume her life as it was before the surgery. She said she wants to walk without a cane and be able to get up and down stairs without pain. Her discharge plans are to return home with services in 1 to 2 weeks. Mary will be followed at the transitional care unit by the physiatrist in charge. Her team will include PT, OT, nursing, nutrition, and social services.

ANALYSIS OF OCCUPATIONAL PERFORMANCE

Mary was evaluated by OT on the day of her admission to the transitional care unit through chart review, interview, observation of her completing functional activity, and assessment of UE motor strength and active range of motion (AROM). She was pleasant and cooperative but needed to be redirected to remain focused. The evaluation revealed no deficits in cognition, perception, sensation, or hearing, but these were not formally tested. She wears glasses at all times. Mary had some decreased AROM in both shoulders, possibly due to the osteoarthritis. Her AROM was at approximately 2/3 range for all shoulder motions. She had no range limitation in the elbows or wrist but could not make a full fist on the left hand without slight pain in the metacarpophalangeal joints. She had a full grasp in the right hand, which is her dominant hand. Mary had 3– strength in the shoulders and 3+ in the elbows and wrists and right hand. Her right hand was stronger than her left hand, but both were functional. Her UE coordination was intact for both gross and fine motor. Mary had pain of 6 of 10 in the left hip only during motion. She had to adhere to total hip precautions and was allowed only partial weight bearing on the affected extremity. Mary did not like to talk about the surgery and would not look at the incision. When

the nurse came in to give her medication and to check on or change the dressing, Mary would either turn and look the other way or close her eyes.

Mary had some slight edema in her left LE. She was at risk for skin breakdown because of the limited motion of her hip and her sleeping position at night. Her bed mobility was fair. She rolled in bed with moderate assistance, bracing herself for pain the whole time. She moved from supine to sit with moderate assistance. She seemed afraid to place any weight on her left leg and performed her transfers slowly and hesitantly. Mary used a standard walker with wheels for her transfers. She transferred from bed to chair with the maximum assistance of one person. She clung tightly to the therapist the entire time and did little to help herself through the transfer. She transferred in a squat-pivot manner instead of a stand-pivot, which she should have been able to do. She performed toilet transfers at the same level of ability. She used a wheelchair for long distances only.

Mary was able to perform her upper body bathing and dressing independently, but in a seated position due to her standing endurance. She was not able to perform her lower body self-care because of her hip precautions. Mary states she was scared to "pop it out" and have to go through "it" again. The occupational therapist attempted to explain the long-handled adaptive equipment to her, but she has declined until "the time is right for my leg." Mary said she is willing to work with OT as long as she does not have to use any "gadgets."

QUESTIONS

Occupations

1. Prioritize the occupations that you would work on. Why did you put them in this order? Did you take Mary's goals into account?

2. What are some of Mary's social and leisure needs? How could Mary's social and leisure needs be met on the unit?

3. Mary had issues with sleep before her surgery. Is this an area that OT should address during her rehabilitation stay? Why or why not?

4. Driving is necessary for Mary. What restrictions, if any, will the surgery have on her ability to drive?

Performance Patterns

5. Identify the roles that have been affected by Mary's surgery and hip replacement.

6. Describe the impact of Mary's surgery on her daily routines as well as on two other key occupations.

7. What personality factors do you feel may affect Mary's performance patterns? In what way?

8. How would you convey to Mary your belief that she did the right thing by having surgery, even though she does not feel that way?

9. Mary is fearful of falling and will not try to do anything on her own. How would you address this fear?

Performance Skills

10. Identify at least 10 key performance skills that have been affected by Mary's current status.

11. How would you have Mary perform her ADL, given her limitations from total hip replacement?

12. What portion of the ADL routine do you anticipate will be most difficult for her to accomplish? How might you adapt this portion of the ADL routine to maximize independence?

13. What do you think Mary's ability to prepare a meal would be? Support your answer with data.

Client Factors

14. What values, beliefs, or spirituality factors do you feel are important to remember when working with Mary? Why? How would you incorporate this information into your intervention?

15. Identify 10 client factors to address during intervention.

16. What interventions would enhance Mary's UE function?

17. Describe preparatory, activity, and occupation intervention methods to address Mary's motor issues.

18. What are posterolateral total hip precautions?

19. Explain these precautions in terms that would be easy for Mary to understand. Write a patient education handout on these precautions.

20. Which devices would be needed for Mary to adhere to total hip precautions while toileting? While sleeping?

21. What feelings do you think Mary might have regarding her recent surgery and why?

22. How might the staff react to Mary's personality? Give two reactions that are positive and two that are not. How can you prevent yourself from responding negatively to Mary?

23. What might be some psychological concerns for Mary when she leaves the transitional care unit?

Contexts and Environment

24. What are some social supports that may be available to Mary?

25. Identify key personal and temporal factors to consider during your OT intervention sessions.

26. If Mary refuses to use the adaptive equipment, what alternatives could you offer to help her reach her goals?

27. What approach might you take to reintroduce the adaptive equipment to Mary to help her reach her goals?

28. What questions would you ask Mary to determine what environmental adaptations might be needed for her safe transition back home?

Theory and Evidence

29. What theory/theories or frame(s) of reference might you use in developing an intervention plan? Describe the rationale for your choices.

30. What, if any, evidence can you find to support your choice of theory/theories and/or frame(s) of reference?

31. What, if any, evidence can you find to support intervention?

Intervention Plan and Goals

32. Write out a problem list for Mary. How would you prioritize these problems for her rehabilitation?

33. Write out a list of Mary's strengths and what you see as barriers to her recovery.

34. What long-term goals would you and Mary set for her OT intervention?

35. What would be appropriate short-term goals for Mary's OT intervention?

36. What are some difficulties that you as a therapist may encounter in helping Mary reach her goals?

37. Write out a specific intervention plan for Mary's first week of intervention, including the frequency of OT sessions. Be prepared to explain why you decided on this plan.

Situations

38. Mary says she will participate in only one group on the unit. Which one do you think would be the most beneficial and why?

39. You enter Mary's room in the morning, and she has gotten a nursing assistant to do all of her self-care for her. What would you say and/or do?

40. You enter Mary's room and find the nursing assistant partly finished with Mary's self-care. What would your reaction be at that time and why?

41. Suppose you overhear Mary talking to her roommate about the therapists at the facility. Mary says that you are a "pain in the butt" for trying to make her use all those "crazy gadgets." What, if anything, would you do?

42. How would it make you feel to know that Mary is annoyed by your attempts to help her?

43. You are in the OT kitchen with Mary practicing making tea. You notice that Mary is not putting any weight on her left LE. "I don't want to take any chances," she says. How do you deal with this?

44. While transferring to the commode, Mary cries out in pain. She says it is her left hip and describes it as a burning pain that shoots down her leg. What would you do?

45. How would you document this incident? Where in the chart would you document it?

Discharge Planning

46. When would you begin discharge planning with Mary?

47. At what level of ability would Mary need to be to return home?

48. What role would Mary's sister play in the discharge process? What role would Mary play?

49. How might Mary continue to work toward her goals once she leaves the unit?

50. Would you recommend continued OT for Mary at home? Why or why not?

51. If you did recommend OT at home, would you still do so if Mary told you she did not want it?

52. If you did not recommend OT at home, what would you want to have in place for Mary to function safely in her home?

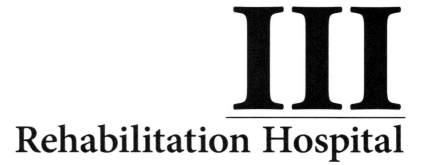

III
Rehabilitation Hospital

Annette: Mechanical Ventilation and Tracheostomy

Kathryn Prizio, MS, OTR/L

OCCUPATIONAL PROFILE

Annette is a 59-year-old woman with no major medical history who presented to an acute care hospital because of weakness, flu-like symptoms, and difficulty breathing that had progressively worsened over a 2- to 3-day period. Before her hospitalization, Annette was completely independent with all mobility and independent with all ADL and IADL. She was driving, working part time as a greeter at a museum, and performing all of the cooking and cleaning at home for herself and her husband. She lives in a split-level home with a bathroom with a tub shower on the top level and a walk-in shower on the first level. Her kitchen, living room, and office are on the first level, and the master bedroom with attached bathroom, two more bedrooms, and a third bathroom are on the upper level. There is an attached garage, which requires one to ascend multiple stairs to get to the main living level. Annette likes to read, knit, and crochet as well as spend time with her adult daughter and two toddler-age grandchildren who live nearby. Annette and her husband often babysit for their grandchildren. She enjoys baking and doing craft activities

with her grandchildren. Annette and her husband have an active social life. They enjoy movies and dining out with friends. Annette was diagnosed in the acute care hospital with diabetic ketoacidosis, left upper lobe pneumonia, and a bacterial infection for which she was started on antibiotics. Her condition worsened with complications of right-sided pneumothorax, atrial fibrillation, and an episode of unresponsiveness that required intubation and mechanical ventilation. There was difficulty weaning her from the ventilator, and therefore she had a tracheostomy placed and a percutaneous endoscopic gastrostomy tube for feeding. She was transferred to a long-term care facility for continued intravenous antibiotics, ventilator weaning, and rehabilitation. Her medical history includes diabetes, asthma, and breast cancer status post-mastectomy 10 years ago. Her goals are to return home and to resume the activities that she was doing before her hospitalization. She would like to manage her home, drive, take care of her grandchildren, and resume her socialization. She will be seen by OT, PT, speech-language pathology, nursing, and social work. Her expected length of stay is 8 to 10 weeks.

Lowenstein NA, Halloran P.
Case Studies Through the Health Care Continuum:
A Workbook for the Occupational Therapy Student, Second Edition (pp 31-34).
© 2015 SLACK Incorporated.

ANALYSIS OF
OCCUPATIONAL PERFORMANCE

The OT evaluation was completed using chart review, interview of patient and husband, observation of functional ADLs, and motor assessment. Documented precautions are nil per os (nothing by mouth [NPO]), no blood pressures to be taken on left UE because of her history of mastectomy, and no blood pressures to be taken on the right UE because of a peripherally inserted central catheter (PICC line) placement. She also has aspiration and "new tracheostomy" precautions (her tracheostomy was inserted less than 1 week ago). OT evaluation revealed that Annette is able to follow simple one-step commands, her AROM is within normal limits for all extremities except for her left shoulder, in which has only 45 degrees of abduction and flexion because of tissue tightness. Manual muscle testing results for right UE are 2–/5 at right shoulder flexion/abduction, 3–/5 elbow flexion/extension, 3–5 wrist flexion/extension, 3–/5 supination/pronation, and 3/5 gross finger flexion/extension; and for left UE: 1/5 shoulder flexion/abduction, 2–/5 elbow flexion/extension, 2+/5 supination/pronation, 2+/5 wrist flexion/extension, and 2+/5 gross finger flexion/extension. Annette is able to wash the lower half of her face and her chest, but otherwise requires total assistance for basic ADL at bed level. She requires maximum assistance of one person for rolling in bed with assist of a second person to manage her ventilator tubing and tracheostomy. She was able to follow two-step commands during bathing assessment.

QUESTIONS

Occupations

1. Identify key occupations that are affected by Annette's condition.

2. Prioritize the occupations in the order you would address them during intervention. Why did you put them in this order? Did you take Annette's goals into account?

Performance Patterns

3. Identify which of Annette's roles are most affected by her current condition.

4. Identify which of Annette's routines are most affected by her current condition.

5. How would this information affect your intervention planning?

6. How would you modify Annette's morning routine during the first week so that she can feel a sense of accomplishment?

7. How would you involve Annette's husband in your interventions?

8. What should Annette's husband learn about Annette's condition?

Performance Skills

9. Identify 10 key performance skills that are strengths for Annette's intervention.

10. Identify 10 key performance skills that have an impact on Annette's ability to participate in her meaningful occupations.

11. Prioritize the performance skills from Question 9 and discuss how the performance skills from Question 10 will influence your intervention.

12. Describe activity- and occupation-based intervention methods to increase Annette's UE strength at bed level.

13. When should you progress Annette to perform ADL at the edge of the bed?

14. Name three occupation-based activities that would help Annette improve her fine motor coordination.

15. What adaptive methods can you think of to assist Annette to communicate with staff and visitors?

Client Factors

16. What values and beliefs do you surmise are important to Annette? How might you use this information during OT intervention?

17. How might you explore her sense of spirituality? Why would this be important?

18. Identify the body functions that are most impaired and need to be addressed initially for intervention.

19. Identify the body functions that remain as strengths for intervention.

20. Describe how you would monitor Annette's vital signs, including heart rate, respiratory rate, and oxygen saturation.

21. Where and how would you take Annette's blood pressure?

22. Is Annette's UE weakness more proximal or more distal?

23. Under what circumstances would you attempt to stand Annette at the edge of the bed?

24. What intervention methods can you use to address Annette's left shoulder deficits?

25. Can Annette lift her left UE against gravity? How do you know this?

26. Describe the "new tracheostomy" precautions.

27. What information does one need to understand in order to work with a PICC line in place?

Contexts and Environment

28. Identify important personal and temporal contexts to consider during Annette's OT assessment and intervention. Why are these important?

29. What social supports, besides her husband, might you explore and how might you use these supports?

30. Would you consider initiating any virtual contexts? If so, which ones and why?

31. What, if any, equipment would you recommend for Annette's home and why?

32. If Annette's insurance does not pay for this equipment and she and her husband cannot afford to pay out of pocket, what alternatives are there?

33. Annette's grandchildren are important to her. How might you use this knowledge in your intervention planning?

34. Annette's husband has never heard of OT and is concerned about your working with her while she is on a ventilator. Write a sample statement of how you would explain your role in Annette's rehabilitation and how you would maintain her safety throughout intervention.

Theory and Evidence

35. What theory/theories or frame(s) of reference might you use in developing an intervention plan? Describe the rationale for your choice(s).

36. What, if any, evidence can you find to support your choice of theory/theories and/or frame(s) of reference?

37. What, if any, evidence can you find to support intervention?

38. What evidence can you find to support OT intervention for patients on ventilators?

Intervention Plan and Goals

39. Because Annette is on a mechanical ventilator, she is unable to speak. How do you think you might assess her cognition? How about her pain? Are there standardized assessments to assess these issues for someone who cannot speak?

40. Would you assess Annette's ability to sit at the edge of the bed? Explain your answer.

41. What role, if any, would an OT assistant have in Annette's OT assessment and intervention?

42. Would you assess Annette's ability to perform self-feeding? Why or why not?

43. Once Annette is able to use a Passy-Muir Valve for communication, are there any standardized assessments that you could use to assess her cognition?

44. How would you assess Annette's fine and gross motor coordination at bed level?

45. During your first week with Annette, what occupations or performance skills would you prioritize for intervention?

46. Write a list of problems for Annette.

47. Write short- and long-term goals for grooming.

48. Write short- and long-term goals for upper body bathing.

Situations

49. After a few days, Annette can be weaned to a tracheostomy mask with a Passy-Muir Valve. Her NPO status is lifted, and speech-language pathology has cleared her for a modified diet. You assess her ability to feed herself at breakfast and find that she is still having some trouble holding the utensils and cutting her food. What adaptive equipment could help Annette to be more independent with self-feeding?

50. The physical therapist asks you to do a "cotreat" with her. Describe how you would collaborate with the physical therapist during a session with Annette. Be specific about the difference between your role as an occupational therapist and the role of the physical therapist. How would you document your session to make it clear you were not doing the same treatment as PT?

51. Annette tells you one day that her left shoulder is "aching." Her pain is anywhere from 5 to 10 out of 10 on the pain scale, and it is waking her up at night. Who do you think you should communicate this to and why?

52. While working with Annette, an alarm on the mechanical ventilator goes off noting that her respiratory rate is 35 breaths per minute, and you notice that her chest is rising and falling more rapidly. What would you do next? Under what circumstances would you continue your intervention session with Annette?

53. You find Annette drinking a coffee that her husband brought her in for her. You know that Annette is supposed to be on a thickened diet and are concerned about aspiration. What should you do? How would you explain to Annette and her husband what it means to be an aspiration risk?

Discharge Planning

54. Annette makes excellent progress after 1 month. She is weaned completely off oxygen, and her tracheostomy is removed. She performs her ADL at sink side and her toileting (with a raised toilet seat and rails) with distant supervision. The PT reports that she can walk more than 200 feet with a rolling walker without difficulty, but uses one because of minor balance issues. Annette continues to have trouble retaining new information in unfamiliar circumstances. The team wants to know if Annette can go home in less than 1 week. Her husband will be able to be with her before and after he goes to work, but she will be alone during the day. What would you need to assess before the team meeting to make a safe recommendation? Would you use a standardized assessment? Which one(s)? Do you have any recommendations for equipment? What IADL do you think you will need to assess before discharge?

55. Would you be recommend home therapy for Annette? Explain your answer.

56. Annette learns that she will have to give herself insulin and will be alone when taking her afternoon pills. How do you see the OT role with Annette's medical management in terms of increasing her independence and also for assessing her ability to safely be discharged home?

8

Frank: Right Cerebrovascular Accident, Left Hemiplegia, Left Neglect

Kathryn Prizio, MS, OTR/L

OCCUPATIONAL PROFILE

Frank is a 68-year-old White man with a diagnosis of right cerebrovascular accident (CVA) of the internal carotid artery with left neglect. In addition, he has coronary artery disease and diabetes. Two weeks ago, Frank was brought to the emergency department by his wife complaining of an unbearable headache, with slurred speech and loss of control on his left side. He was admitted to the acute care hospital and was stabilized; after 5 days, he was transferred to the rehabilitation hospital for more extensive rehabilitation.

Before his CVA, Frank had been a very active man. He recently retired from his job as a postal worker and is looking forward to traveling with his wife and tending to his garden. He is an avid gardener and woodworker and anticipates enjoying his two hobbies more extensively.

Frank has a son from a previous marriage who does not live nearby and with whom he has a strained relationship. Frank and his wife live in a ranch-style home in a suburban neighborhood. There are five steps into the front door, and the garage is not attached to the house. They are friendly with some of their neighbors, but others are new to the neighborhood and they do not know them well. Frank has always done all the maintenance tasks on his home. Frank's wife does the meal preparation and laundry. Frank will sometimes do the grocery shopping or go with his wife on this errand. He makes his own breakfast and lunch if his wife is not at home.

Frank has many friends from the post office, and he has maintained his weekly bowling night with them after retirement. He and his wife have a strong marriage. They are planning on his return home after his discharge from the rehabilitation hospital. Their goal is for him to return home and resume his hobbies. He looks forward to picking up his life where it was before it was disrupted by the CVA. Frank's wife is supportive of these goals and will do whatever it takes to get him home to live life as before.

He will be seen by OT, PT, speech therapy, and recreational therapy. He will also be seen by nursing, dietary, and physiatry. His expected length of stay is 3 weeks.

Lowenstein NA, Halloran P.
Case Studies Through the Health Care Continuum: A Workbook for the Occupational Therapy Student, Second Edition (pp 35-38).
© 2015 SLACK Incorporated.

Analysis of Occupational Performance

OT evaluation took place over two intervention sessions through observation, interview, manual muscle testing, perceptual and sensory testing, and the Barthel Index of ADLs (Mahoney & Barthel, 1965), on which Frank scored a 10 of 20. He has no deficits in his hearing or vision, aside from wearing glasses for distance. He does have deficits in perception, with difficulty in figure–ground and spatial relations. He demonstrates right–left confusion and a profound left neglect. Observation of Frank completing his daily routine showed cognitive deficits, including poor attention span, insight, judgment, and safety awareness. He has difficulty maneuvering around his room and the hospital environment and is constantly bumping into things on the left side. Sensation testing finds impaired sensation for light touch and sharp–dull, as well as impaired stereognosis on his affected side.

Frank has no AROM or sensory deficits in his right UE. He is right-handed. He presents with weakness in his left UE and LE, has poor dynamic sitting and standing balance, and his static standing balance is fair with good static sitting balance. His PROM in his left UE is shoulder flexion to 85 degrees, abduction to 70 degrees, and elbow flexion to 100 degrees. His wrist and hand have PROM within normal limits (WNL), but he has muscle tone of 2 on the Asworth Scale in his fingers and wrist. He presents with tone of 2 on the Ashworth Scale throughout the UE, neck, and trunk, and 1 on the Ashworth Scale in his LE. His left UE has AROM as follows: shoulder flexion/extension: 0 to 50 degrees; adduction/abduction: 0 to 45 degrees; internal rotation: 0 to 5 degrees; external rotation: 0 to 15 degrees; elbow flexion/extension: 0 to 60; supination: 0 to 15 degrees; pronation: WNL; wrist extension: 0 to 10 degrees; wrist flexion: 0 to 45 degrees; finger flexion: half normal range. His finger extension is weak. He is unable to release objects. His strength is not being tested because of his increased tone. Coordination on the left is impaired for both fine and gross motor.

During the ADL evaluation, Frank demonstrates difficulty with right–left discrimination. He has a great deal of difficulty managing his clothing. He is unable to figure out the front from the back or the sleeve hole from the neck hole and needs maximum assistance with all dressing tasks. He appears to have a dressing apraxia. Bathing was completed while sitting at the sink. He neglected his left side completely, did not attend to objects on the left side of the sink, and needed a great deal of verbal cueing and physical guidance to complete the task.

He ambulates with a hemi walker and minimum assist because of his poor balance. He transfers with minimum assist and moderate verbal cueing because of poor safety awareness.

Frank is amiable and likes the staff members. He teases them and is good at involving humor in interactions with others. He does not understand why he needs so much therapy or why he has to be in the rehabilitation hospital. His wife told him that the doctor said he needed to be here and that is why he stays.

Questions

Occupations

1. What areas of occupation would you address during Frank's rehabilitation stay? How would you prioritize these? Did you consider Frank's wishes in this list?

2. What would you identify as the self-care deficits most likely to have an impact on his rehabilitation in the area of bathing and dressing? Why are these obstacles for Frank?

3. Knowing Frank's hobbies and interests, would you be able to incorporate any of these into your intervention sessions? How would you go about this?

Performance Patterns

4. Identify key roles that Frank had before his CVA. What impact do you see his CVA having on these roles?

5. Describe ways in which OT may assist Frank in returning to some of these roles.

6. Identify key routines that Frank had before his CVA. What impact do you see his CVA having on these routines?

7. Describe ways in which OT may assist Frank in resuming some of these routines.

Performance Skills

8. Identify 10 key performance skills that are negatively affected by Frank's CVA.

9. Identify 10 key performance skills that are strengths. How might these strengths be utilized during intervention?

10. How would you set up Frank to bathe at the sink? What kind of physical and verbal cueing do you anticipate he might need and how much?

11. Would you give Frank adaptive equipment for his ADL? Why or why not? If you would, what kind would you give him?

12. How would you address Frank's left neglect during his ADL? What type of intervention activities would you use, and how would you set up his environment? Can

you think of activities outside of the ADL routine to use as well?

13. How would you address Frank's dressing apraxia?

14. Create an instruction sheet for Frank to follow for his morning ADL routine.

15. Frank used to make his wife her morning coffee and breakfast of toast and cereal. Would this be a good intervention activity to do with Frank? Why or why not?

16. You decide to do a kitchen activity with Frank. What safety measures would you want to follow?

17. What considerations and staff education would you have in setting up Frank's room so that he can use the television remote, call bell, and urinal, and find other items on his bedside table?

Client Factors

18. Identify and prioritize Frank's neurological deficits.

19. What intervention activities would you use to reduce the muscle tone in Frank's UE and trunk?

20. How would you incorporate purposeful activity into your intervention plan?

21. Would you fabricate a splint for Frank's UE? If so, why and what type? What would the wearing schedule be? If you would not use a splint for Frank, explain the reasoning behind your decision.

22. In what ways will Frank's cognitive and perceptual deficits affect his daily functioning?

23. What functional activities would you use to address Frank's cognitive and perceptual deficits?

24. What preparatory, activity, and/or occupation-based intervention methods would you use to address Frank's cognitive and perceptual deficits?

25. What are the primary safety concerns that should be addressed with Frank? How would you and the team address these concerns?

26. What are some ways to support Frank psychologically to help him deal with his decreased abilities?

Contexts and Environment

27. What type of adaptations to the environment or adaptive equipment would you want to use in addressing the safety concerns identified in Question 25?

28. Would Frank be a good candidate for using a tablet or other assistive device to help him resume ADL? Why or why not?

29. Frank uses humor throughout his intervention sessions, especially when he is having a particularly difficult time with something. Why do you think he is always trying to be funny, and how would you deal with it?

30. What concerns might Frank have relating to his loss of function?

31. Would you include Frank's wife in any patient/family education? If so, in what areas?

32. Using the areas identified in Question 31, how would you go about educating Frank and his wife?

33. How would you work with the team to educate Frank on safety issues?

34. What social supports can you identify, and how might you incorporate them into your intervention?

Theory and Evidence

35. What theory/theories or frame(s) of reference might you use in developing an intervention plan? Describe the rationale for your choice(s).

36. What, if any, evidence can you find to support your choice of theory/theories and/or frame(s) of reference?

37. What theory/theories and/or frame(s) of reference would you use to remediate Frank's neuromusculoskeletal deficits? Why? Can you find evidence to support the use of this for intervention?

Intervention Plan and Goals

38. Write out a problem list for Frank.

39. What are Frank's strengths, and how could these be drawn on during your intervention planning?

40. Identify at least two functional assessments to evaluate Frank's LE and UE use. Why did you choose these? What information will they provide to assist in intervention planning?

41. What would the long-term goals be, given what you know about what Frank and his wife want? How would you incorporate Frank's wishes into your intervention planning?

42. What are your short-term goals for Frank?

43. If you think that Frank and his wife have unrealistic long-term goals for his rehab stay, how would you handle this?

44. What obstacles do you see to Frank reaching his stated goals?

45. What role would a COTA assistant play in Frank's assessment and intervention? Be specific in terms of

skills during evaluation, intervention planning, and intervention sessions.

46. Are there other standardized assessments that you would administer? For what areas? Why did you select the assessments and what information would you hope to gain from them?

47. Did you choose assessments at the client factors–body function level or participation level, or were they occupation-based? Find an assessment that targets a different level (body function, participation, occupation).

Situations

48. Frank has regained AROM of 15 degrees in all motions of his UE. How would the intervention plan be modified? How would this affect his ability to use his UE functionally during ADLs and other activities?

49. You walk into Frank's room in the morning to work with him on ADLs and find him in bed with the bedrails up, but trying to climb over them. He already has one leg over the bedrail and is trying to get his left leg over now. What would you do and why?

50. During an intervention session in the OT kitchen, Frank is making a cup of instant coffee. He turns on the stove, gets the kettle, and takes it to the sink to fill. He starts the water, notices a sponge, and starts to clean up the area around the sink, the sink itself, and the outside of the cabinets around the sink. He has forgotten the stove and the kettle and has left the water running for 5 minutes during his cleaning. What do you think is the cause of this behavior, and how would you refocus Frank? Would you adjust future kitchen activities and, if so, how?

51. Frank is in the middle of dressing himself. He has been following a set of cards with the steps for dressing on

them with good results. Today, Frank is not attending to the cards. He starts to get up to leave the room, but only has his boxers on; how would you redirect Frank to his dressing task?

52. During functional mobility, Frank has progressed to ambulating with the hemi walker and supervision. However, he bumps into objects on his left side (the door frame, the bed, the dresser). How would you address this during your intervention sessions?

Discharge Planning

53. Frank is being discharged home. He now requires supervision for dressing and bathing using his cue cards and equipment. He continues to be impulsive and has poor insight into his deficits, and the carryover of new learning requires frequent repetitions. He can use his left UE to stabilize objects, but gross- and fine-motor coordination are still poor. He continues to have left neglect and has difficulty compensating for it. What services would you recommend for Frank and why?

54. Write a referral on Frank for the home care agency that will be seeing him next.

55. What discharge instructions would you give Frank's wife?

REFERENCE

Mahoney, F. I., & Barthel, D. (1965). Functional evaluation: The Barthel Index. *Maryland State Med Journal, 14,* 56-61. Retrieved from http://www.strokecenter.org/wp-content/uploads/2011/08/barthel.pdf

9

Geri: Status Post Pneumonia

Kathryn Prizio, MS, OTR/L

Occupational Profile

Geri is a 74-year-old woman who presented to her primary care physician with complaints of viral cold symptoms, including a runny nose, sinus congestion, a sore throat, coughing, and shortness of breath. Her doctor found that her oxygen saturation was in the 80s and recommended that she be admitted to an acute care hospital. In the emergency department, a chest x-ray confirmed right lower lobe pneumonia for which she was treated with intravenous antibiotics. She was also treated with intravenous steroids, a nebulizer, and supplemental oxygen for chronic obstructive pulmonary disease (COPD) exacerbation. She was stabilized and then transferred to a rehabilitation hospital for continued medical management and rehabilitation. She was diagnosed with COPD 5 years ago but has never needed oxygen until now. Geri has also been dealing with fibromyalgia for 10 years.

Geri is a retired certified nursing assistant, and she and her husband have been married for 26 years. They have no children. They live in a two-story home; however, before her admission to the acute care hospital, she was staying on the first floor because of increasing shortness of breath.

She spends nights sleeping on the sofa because it is so difficult for her to climb the stairs. Geri is independent with functional ambulation of short distances in her home and independent with her basic ADLs, although her husband points out that on "bad days" she does not wash or get dressed anymore. Sleeping on the sofa exacerbates her chronic pain syndrome and so she does not feel like doing anything else for the rest of the day. She spends most of her time being inactive and watching TV. She and her husband used to enjoy going out for dinner and going for rides to the beach; however, she has had no energy for the past few months. Geri also used to enjoy grocery shopping, cooking, and cleaning, but she has had to rely on her husband to do these tasks for the past few months. She does not see her friends because she is too tired to go out with them when they call her. Geri still smokes; she says she would like to quit, but needs a cigarette to help her relax. Geri says she smokes only two or three cigarettes a day. She is being seen by OT and PT during her stay at the rehabilitation hospital. Her stay is expected to last 4 weeks. Geri's goal is to return home and to be able to sleep in the bed with her husband and to be able to resume her IADLs and community outings. Geri has Medicare Part A and B.

Lowenstein NA, Halloran P.
Case Studies Through the Health Care Continuum:
A Workbook for the Occupational Therapy Student, Second Edition (pp 39-41).
© 2015 SLACK Incorporated.

ANALYSIS OF OCCUPATIONAL PERFORMANCE

OT evaluation was completed through observation, functional tasks, and motor assessments. The results of these assessments reveal that Geri does not appear to have any cognitive, sensory, or visual perceptual deficits. She has good memory and good overall judgment and safety during functional activity. Her UE AROM and upper body strength are within functional limits; however, she is unable to comb her hair because of increased shortness of breath. Geri is able to wash her upper body and independently put on her shirt, but she requires help to stand to wash her bottom and don her pants and socks because of increased shortness of breath. Additionally, after standing to pull up her pants, her oxygen saturation decreases from 94% to 86% while on 2 liters of oxygen via nasal cannula. She is able to transfer to a manual wheelchair with minimal assistance; however, she is still using the bedpan because it is "too hard" for her to walk to the bathroom. Geri expresses currently feeling "depressed" and scared. She states she is willing to participate with OT because she hopes it will help her to "feel normal again." Geri has a tub/shower and low toilets in both her upstairs and downstairs bathrooms. She states that getting up from her toilets has been "more of a struggle" lately. The admitting doctor has ordered that she be on 2 liters of oxygen by nasal cannula to keep her oxygen saturation greater than 95% during functional activity.

QUESTIONS

Occupations

1. Identify all of the occupations that are affected by Geri's COPD.

2. Prioritize these occupations from Geri's point of view and from your point of view as her clinician. Are the lists different? What considerations did you take into account to create your list?

Performance Patterns

3. Identify key roles that Geri has given up.

4. Which of these roles do you feel Geri could resume after discharge home? Why? Would your OT intervention target these roles directly or indirectly? Explain.

5. What new routines would Geri need to develop after discharge home? Why? How would your OT intervention target these routines? Explain.

Performance Skills

6. Identify 10 key performance skills that may be negatively affecting Geri.

7. Identify 10 key performance skills that may be strengths to consider when developing and implementing your intervention plan.

8. How would these 20 performance skills influence your OT intervention?

9. Describe an intervention to assist Geri to be more independent with toileting given that she is currently too scared to walk to the bathroom.

10. What strategies would you use to help Geri to be more independent with lower body dressing?

11. Suggest nonpharmacologic pain management strategies for managing Geri's fibromyalgia symptoms.

Client Factors

12. Identify 10 key body functions that may be barriers for Geri's optimal occupational functioning.

13. Identify 10 key body functions that may be supports to achieving Geri's optimal occupational functioning.

14. Describe three energy conservation techniques you could teach Geri to use when cooking.

15. What values and beliefs might influence Geri's motivation for OT? Why?

16. How would you explain to Geri how to use a perceived rate of exertion scale.

Contexts and Environment

17. Identify key personal and temporal contexts to consider during assessment and intervention.

18. Identify social supports that Geri and her husband might utilize.

19. What are some physical barriers in her home? How would you recommend they address these?

20. What precautions do Geri and her husband need to learn regarding being on supplemental oxygen?

21. What, if any, equipment would you recommend for Geri's home? Why?

22. What is the cost of this equipment? Does her insurance pay for it?

Theory and Evidence

23. What theory/theories or frame(s) of reference might you use in developing an intervention plan? Describe the rationale for your choice(s).

24. What, if any, evidence can you find to support your choice(s) of theory/theories and/or frame(s) of reference?

25. What, if any, evidence can you find to support intervention?

Intervention Plan and Goals

26. Identify strengths and barriers that may have an impact on your intervention with Geri.

27. Suggest three long-term goals and corresponding short-term goals for Geri's 4-week stay.

28. Describe methods for objectively measuring and documenting Geri's pain before, during, and after intervention sessions.

29. Would you want to complete any other standardized assessments? If so, are these occupation or body-function based?

30. What tasks would you assign to an OT assistant for assessment and intervention? Why?

Situations

31. During your first intervention session, Geri's oxygen saturation decreases to 80% while transferring to the commode on 2 liters of oxygen via nasal cannula. To whom do you think you should communicate this information and why? What is your immediate response to this change during your intervention session?

32. As Geri's hospitalization progresses, you learn that she is going to require supplemental oxygen when she goes home. What would your immediate safety concerns be? What else would you want to know?

33. During your intervention session, Geri demonstrates increased shortness of breath while standing at the sink to brush her teeth and states, "I can't breathe." What should you do next? How could you determine if it is safe to progress with intervention?

34. You determine that it is safe to progress with intervention. How might you modify the task of brushing her teeth?

35. During a meal preparation session, you note that Geri is having difficulty in properly sequencing the steps for making a familiar cookie recipe. Would you consider formally assessing her cognitive status? If so, what standardized assessment would you use?

Discharge Planning

36. What are some options for Geri improving her sleeping comfort if she is unable to climb stairs before discharge home?

37. Geri's husband notes that Geri gets fatigued after walking 2 or 3 minutes with a standard rolling walker. He wants to know the safest way to get Geri to her appointments and to take her places in the community. Write a sample statement of your recommendations.

38. Assume that you are going to recommend home OT services for Geri. Write a justification based on the deficits that have been noted thus far.

10

Harris: Spinal Cord Injury— T3 Incomplete

OCCUPATIONAL PROFILE

Harris is a 22-year-old Black man with a diagnosis of incomplete spinal cord injury at T3 and resultant paraplegia due to an auto accident. Harris also fractured his right tibia and fibula and right proximal radius and ulna in the accident. Harris was admitted to the rehabilitation hospital from the acute care hospital where he stayed for 2.5 weeks after his accident.

Harris lives with his fiancée, Marsha, on the 15th floor of a new apartment complex in the city. It is a small one-bedroom apartment. They intend to be married after his graduation from college. Harris has one more semester to complete for his baccalaureate degree in computer science. He also works full time for his brother's plumbing business as a bookkeeper—work that he can do on his computer at home or at his brother's office (which is in his brother's home). His brother lives 5 miles away by car, in a home that has six steps at the entrance and no ramp. During the little free time he has, Harris likes to travel with Marsha and golf with his friends. They like to entertain and enjoy going to the movies for their weekly date night. Marsha works as a dental hygienist at a busy dental practice. Harris had no functional deficits before the accident.

Harris's family is extremely supportive and visits daily. His brother, Jeff, calls frequently, and his mother cooks his favorite meals, which she brings in for the nurses as well as for Harris. Harris's father is not well and cannot visit as often because of respiratory distress, but he telephones his son regularly. Marsha has taken time off work to be with Harris every day at the rehabilitation hospital. She wants to be involved in learning as much as she can to help Harris "get better."

Harris was admitted to the rehabilitation hospital with the goal of returning home, finishing his degree, and graduating on time (in 4 months). He is eager to get started and tells the admission nurse "the more therapy, the better." Harris will be evaluated by PT, OT, nursing, social work, and the physiatrist.

Lowenstein NA, Halloran P.
Case Studies Through the Health Care Continuum:
A Workbook for the Occupational Therapy Student, Second Edition (pp 43-46).
© 2015 SLACK Incorporated.

Analysis of Occupational Performance

Harris was evaluated with observation, functional activities, chart review, sensory testing, manual muscle testing, and goniometry. Upon evaluation, he was talkative and motivated. He is in a wheelchair with lateral supports. His right UE is in a full-arm cast, and his right LE is in an Aircast from the toes to the knee. Harris is right-handed. When asked how he has been feeling since the accident, his reply is "fine." When the question is rephrased as to his emotional state, his response is the same.

Harris has no cognitive, perceptual, visual, or hearing deficits. He has no sensation in either LE and reports no sensation in his buttocks either. His UE sensation is intact, as is the sensation in his superior trunk region. His sensation is impaired in his inferior trunk region. Harris's low back area could not be assessed during the evaluation because of his position in the chair.

Harris has no AROM in the LEs. His motion is intact in the left UE and cervical area. His right UE cannot be fully assessed because of the cast. Motion in his right digits is normal, given the limitations of the cast. His left UE has normal strength; right UE has not been fully assessed, but Harris can lift this arm up over his head even with the cast.

Harris has no complaints of pain except for stiffness in his neck. He has some slight edema in the right digits at the metacarpophalangeal to distal interphalangeal joints but no cyanosis. He has multiple bruises and abrasions over his body that nursing is monitoring. Harris's unsupported sitting balance is poor to fair and he is unable to sit up independently without minimal assistance or lateral supports. He does attempt to correct himself when leaning, but lacks the strength to maintain upright posture without external assistance. He is independent in sitting with the lateral supports in the wheelchair.

Harris uses a sliding board with moderate assistance to transfer from surface to surface. He is nonambulatory and non–weight-bearing on the right leg. Harris requires occasional assistance to propel himself in a wheelchair because of his inability to use his right arm. He can perform bathing tasks sitting in front of the sink in his wheelchair and can wash his face, hands, and chest with setup. He requires total assistance for back, buttocks, and legs. He requires maximum assistance for dressing himself. Harris reports feeding himself without help, although "it's messy sometimes." Harris has a catheter for urination and had been incontinent of bowel since the accident. His admission Functional Independence Measure (FIM; Uniform Data System for Medical Rehabilitation) scores were 37 of 91 on the motor subscale and 35 of 35 on the cognition subscale.

Harris wants to get started with therapy right away. He says his goals for rehabilitation are to "walk out of here and get on with my life." His expected length of stay is 6 weeks. His automobile insurance is covering his medical expenses, with a cap of $500,000.

Questions

Occupations

1. What are some of the occupations that you would immediately address with Harris? Why did you choose these occupations, and how would working on these help meet Harris's goals?

2. Explain how you would set up an ADL session with Harris.

3. Harris's brother has told him not to worry about his job, but Harris keeps talking about it. Would you incorporate this into the intervention plan? If so, how?

4. Harris keeps talking about not wanting to miss any of his classes or course material. Do you think it is realistic for him to expect to graduate on time? What would you convey to Harris in regard to this goal? Could OT support him in this area? If so, what would you do to support his goal?

Performance Patterns

5. What roles have been most disrupted by Harris's spinal cord injury? How might you address some of these during your interventions?

6. What are some of your safety concerns for Harris given his condition?

7. What type of education should Harris and his family receive regarding spinal cord injuries at the thoracic level?

8. What skills will Harris need to learn to incorporate into his daily routine to prevent self-injury?

9. Find three agencies in your area that provide services for individuals with spinal cord injuries.

Performance Skills

10. Identify 10 key performance skills that may have a negative impact on Harris.

11. Identify 10 key performance skills that may be strengths to consider when developing and implementing your intervention plan.

12. How will these 20 performance skills influence your OT intervention?

Client Factors

13. Given that Harris has an incomplete spinal cord injury, what might you expect to see with regard to his muscle function?

14. Describe an intervention session focused on Harris's balance deficits.

15. Describe an intervention session focused on Harris's UE status while the cast is on his right arm.

16. Describe your UE intervention focus once the cast is removed at 8 weeks postinjury. Would you use preparatory, activity, or occupation-based intervention methods? Why did you choose the methods that you did?

17. Create an activity or occupation-based method for working on improving Harris's sitting balance out of the chair.

18. PT would like to cotreat with you for Harris's afternoon session. Describe what might be accomplished by having a cotreatment session with PT.

19. Describe interventions that could occur in a session cotreating with PT. How would you ensure that you are not duplicating services, and how would you document differently from PT?

20. Why is Harris's LE status important to you as his occupational therapist?

21. How does Harris appear to be coping with the accident and his injury?

22. What might be the impact of his accident on his relationship with his family?

23. What new issues will Harris's injury bring to his future with Marsha?

24. Even though Harris is not expressing such concerns, should they be addressed? If so, by whom?

Contexts and Environment

25. Identify personal and temporal factors to consider for assessment and intervention. Why are these important?

26. Identify social supports, other than Marsha. How would you incorporate these into your intervention planning?

27. Would you recommend any virtual adaptations? If so, what and why?

28. What type of adaptive equipment might help Harris to be more independent while at the hospital?

29. What type of adaptive equipment might Harris need to function optimally at home?

30. What equipment would you order for Harris's apartment?

31. What type of teaching would need to be done with Marsha before Harris goes home?

32. What type of wheelchair would you and the PT order for Harris to take home? Be specific and include cost and payer source.

Theory and Evidence

33. What theory/theories or frame(s) of reference might you use in developing an intervention plan? Describe the rationale for your choice(s).

34. What, if any, evidence can you find to support your choice(s) of theory/theories and/or frame(s) of reference?

35. What, if any, evidence can you find to support intervention?

Intervention Plan and Goals

36. What are your first thoughts when you hear Harris's own goals for his rehabilitation stay? What would you say in response?

37. Write a list of problem areas you feel would need to be addressed for Harris to achieve his goals.

38. What do you see as Harris's strengths to reaching these goals? What are the barriers?

39. How could you incorporate his strengths into the intervention plan to help him meet his goals?

40. What long-term goals would you and Harris set for OT intervention?

41. What short-term goals would you and Harris set for OT intervention?

42. How would your goals and/or intervention plan change for his ADL training once the casts are removed?

Situations

43. You are working with Harris in a cotreatment session with PT. Harris still has no AROM in his LEs, but has improved in his sitting balance and trunk strength. Harris asks the PT when she thinks he'll walk. The PT acts like she does not hear him, and he turns to you with the question. What would you say?

44. You see Harris in his room trying to do sit-ups in his bed. He is unable to do them, which only seems to make him try harder. What would you do in response to seeing this?

45. Harris's friends from work come to visit him as he is ending an OT session. They start lifting the weights in the gym and showing off to one another. How might this make Harris feel? What would you say?

46. During an ADL session with Harris, you notice a small sore in the gluteal fold. What could be done to treat this problem? Why might it have occurred in the first place?

47. The doctor has cleared Harris to weight-bear on his LEs. The PT wants to try the tilt table and asks you to help. Harris is excited and calls Marsha at home to come see him. Marsha arrives at the hospital while Harris is strapped onto the table in an upright position. She tries to be positive, but starts to cry. Harris demands to be put back in the chair and is obviously shaken by her reaction. What would you do and say to Marsha? To Harris? To the team?

48. Harris continues to show improvement through his determination. He is performing the sliding board transfers and ADL in bed independently. He wants to be able to shower alone. How could you help him achieve this goal? Explain.

49. His catheter has been removed, but Harris still is not continent all the time because of motor and sensory loss. What could you do to help Harris achieve his goals of continence?

50. You wanted to work on Harris's UE strength by having him play a card game with weights on his wrist. Harris refuses to participate, stating, "I'm here for work, not games." What are your thoughts about this statement, and what do you do?

Discharge Planning

51. Harris plans to go home soon. What questions should you ask him to assist with the transition back to the community?

52. Harris wants to return to work. How long do you think it will be before he is able to do that? What adaptations need to be in place before Harris returns to work?

53. Harris has also spoken of returning to school because he has only one semester left. What will he need to investigate before his return to the college?

54. What resources might there be at the college to support Harris's return to his academics?

55. Harris is going to continue with rehabilitation through the Visiting Nurse Association until he can arrange outpatient treatment. What would you recommend the home OT work on?

11

Ingrid: Traumatic Brain Injury (Rancho Los Amigos Level V)

OCCUPATIONAL PROFILE

Ingrid is a 45-year-old White woman who suffered a traumatic brain injury (TBI) from a skiing accident. She had been on a skiing vacation in the Northwest with her husband and two children—a 15-year-old son and an 8-year-old daughter. Ingrid lost control and tumbled several hundred feet down the mountain before hitting a tree and coming to a stop. During the tumble, her head hit the ground several times. She was wearing a helmet, but the number of times her head hit the ground and the icy conditions caused her to sustain a TBI. The ski patrol arrived at the scene within 10 minutes and found Ingrid unconscious. She was transported to the local hospital where she was stabilized and then taken by helicopter to a large hospital that could deal with her head trauma. She spent several weeks in the acute care hospital, which was near the ski resort, several hundred miles from her home. She was discharged to a rehabilitation hospital in the same city as the acute care hospital for further therapy. Her husband is staying in a nearby hotel, and their children were sent home; Ingrid's parents are living with them in their home.

Before the accident, Ingrid was a social worker in a skilled nursing facility. She had no deficits in any occupational performance area. She was active in her daughter's school, volunteering to help out with reading in the classroom and on other school committees. She and her family live in a two-story colonial home in a suburban neighborhood. Her husband, Tom, works as an accountant for a small accounting firm. He has taken time off from work to stay near Ingrid's hospital, which was far from the family's home, so that she does not feel abandoned and alone. Although Tom does not want to leave Ingrid alone in the rehabilitation hospital, he is afraid to take more time off from work. The family needs the income and health benefits, and the tax season is approaching. Their financial situation will be tight without Ingrid's income. Ingrid is religious and attended church each week. She took her children with her, but Tom did not participate. The family enjoyed taking vacations together, and usually these centered around such activities as skiing, hiking, and snorkeling. Both Tom and Ingrid felt that the kids were more likely to want to come on these trips and enjoy them. Ingrid and Tom met in college and have kept in touch with many of their college friends, although they are scattered around the country. They like to watch movies, cook meals, and take walks together when they are not busy shuffling their children to different activities.

Lowenstein NA, Halloran P.
Case Studies Through the Health Care Continuum:
A Workbook for the Occupational Therapy Student, Second Edition (pp 47-50).
© 2015 SLACK Incorporated.

The plan is that Ingrid will be discharged to her home in 6 weeks. She is being seen by OT, PT, speech therapy, social work, nursing, psychologist, and physiatrist.

ANALYSIS OF OCCUPATIONAL PERFORMANCE

OT evaluation was completed using chart review, observation of Ingrid's completing morning routine, manual muscle testing, and the Rancho Los Amigos Scale of Cognitive Functioning, on which Ingrid was identified as a Level V—confused, inappropriate, nonagitated. She responds to simple directions, but is highly distractible and has poor memory. Her verbal skills are also impaired, with some automatic social conversations possible. She has intact sensation, vision, and hearing. Perceptual processing is impaired for spatial relations, categorization, and position in space.

Her physical status presents with tone of 2 on the Ashworth Scale in her UEs, with the left side somewhat worse than the right. She has PROM in the left shoulder of 0 to 85 degrees flexion, 0 to 50 degrees external rotation, and 0 to 80 degrees internal rotation. Her UE PROM in the right shoulder is 0 to 105 degrees flexion, 0 to 70 degrees external rotation, 0 to 80 degrees internal rotation, 0 to 40 degrees horizontal abduction, and 0 to 90 degrees horizontal adduction. PROM in remainder is within functional limits. AROM is less than half normal AROM in both shoulders. She also has muscle tone of 1 on the Ashworth Scale in her trunk and 2 in her LEs. She continues to demonstrate some primitive reflexes, especially asymmetrical tonic neck reflex, and she has decreased equilibrium and righting reactions. Her coordination is impaired due to the tone in her UEs. Ingrid is right-handed.

Ingrid requires minimum physical assistance and frequent verbal cues for all transfers and wheelchair mobility. She is currently nonambulatory. She requires moderate assistance with all ADL tasks because of her physical and cognitive deficits. Ingrid currently has little insight into her deficits. She has photos of her children in her room and can identify them with cueing. She initially did not recognize her husband, Tom, and kept calling him "doctor," but she has recently begun to recognize him as her husband. She has expressed anger at the staff and feels she is being kept a prisoner against her wishes. She lacks initiation and, when in a group situation, says whatever is on her mind, even if it is a criticism of another patient or staff member. She has alienated a few staff members and patients by calling them "fat," "stupid," or "ugly," among other things.

When asked what her goals are, Ingrid only states, "eat breakfast and drive a pie." Tom is hopeful that Ingrid can improve enough to return home, drive, and take care of the kids. Ingrid has disability insurance from her job, but it does not cover all of her medical expenses or make up entirely for her lost salary.

QUESTIONS

Occupations

1. Identify all of the occupations that are affected by Ingrid's TBI. How would your prioritize these in terms of intervention, taking Tom's goals into account?

2. Describe how the occupation of community mobility will affect her children and Tom.

3. What types of simple home-management tasks would you start to work on with Ingrid?

4. What types of leisure activities would you try with Ingrid, and why did you choose these?

Performance Patterns

5. What roles are most affected by Ingrid's TBI? Which of these do you feel have the most impact on others? Why?

6. How important will establishing routines be for Ingrid's recovery? Why?

7. Describe the intervention techniques that you would use to establish a morning ADL routine that Ingrid could learn to do with supervision.

8. Describe ways you could use spiritual performance patterns during your intervention.

Performance Skills

9. Identify five (in each area) primary motor, process, and social interaction skills that have been affected by Ingrid's TBI. Why did you identify these as the primary skills in each area?

10. Ingrid is able to brush her teeth and wash her hands and face at the sink from the wheelchair with setup. What would you address next in the bathing/grooming performance area? How would you go about this?

11. Would you teach Ingrid to use adaptive equipment for her ADL routine? Explain your answer.

12. You want to do a kitchen activity with Ingrid. What activity would you choose, and how would you organize it to ensure her success?

13. During your kitchen activity, what safety concerns would you have? Why? How would you handle these during your intervention to ensure Ingrid's safety?

14. How would you collaborate with other staff members in addressing Ingrid's safety issues?

15. What other standardized assessments would you administer? why did you choose these? Are any of them occupation based or activity based?

Client Factors

16. Identify important values and beliefs that may influence your OT intervention.

17. In what way might Ingrid's spirituality influence her response to her accident? How might spirituality influence her children's response?

18. Ingrid's coordination is impaired for gross- and fine-motor activities. Address her sitting position and explain why correct sitting position is an important component for coordination.

19. After you positioned Ingrid correctly, what techniques would you use to normalize her muscle tone, and with what areas of her UE would you start?

20. Describe preparatory, activity-based, and occupation-centered intervention activities that you would use to help normalize muscle tone.

21. PT and OT work closely in the area of normalizing muscle tone. How would you ensure that your intervention is different from PT's intervention?

22. Given Ingrid's Rancho Los Amigos level, what types of interventions (preparatory methods/tasks, activity-based, and occupation-centered) would you do to work on her cognitive deficits?

23. From what type of structure, if any, would Ingrid benefit to compensate for her cognitive deficits?

24. Given Ingrid's perceptual problems, what key areas would you expect to be the most affected and why?

25. Ingrid gets easily frustrated during her intervention sessions. How would you deal with this issue?

Contexts and Environment

26. Identify key personal and temporal contexts to consider for assessment and intervention.

27. Tom is looking toward the day when Ingrid returns home. What environmental modifications, either temporary or permanent, would you suggest he make knowing the type of home they live in?

28. What type of modifications might you need to make to Ingrid's wheelchair, and what pieces of adaptive equipment would you give to her so that she can carry her memory aids?

29. What support services exist in Ingrid's community for patients and families with TBI? Which one might Ingrid benefit from and why?

30. Describe social supports that will assist the family when she returns home. In what ways would you suggest they utilize these?

Theory and Evidence

31. What theory or frame of reference would you use to address Ingrid's motor issues? Why did you choose this one? Is there evidence to support the use of this theory/frame of reference for individuals with TBI?

32. What other theory/theories or frame(s) of reference might you use in developing an intervention plan? Describe the rationale for your choice(s).

Interventions Plan and Goals

33. Write a list of problems that would need to be addressed by OT during Ingrid's expected rehab stay of 6 weeks.

34. Prioritize the problems to be addressed based on Ingrid's and Tom's goals.

35. What are Ingrid's strengths? What are some of the challenges she would bring to your intervention?

36. Based on the problem list from Question 33, write a list of long- and short-term goals.

37. Given Ingrid's level of cognitive function, how would you make your goals client centered?

38. How would you include Ingrid's husband in your intervention plan?

39. What role would other team members have in meeting Ingrid's rehab needs? What role would a COTA have in assessment and intervention?

Situations

40. Ingrid is taking a shower for the first time with OT. She is very distractible and has a short attention span and little insight. How would you structure the task so that it is successful and not frustrating for her?

41. Ingrid has always worn tailored clothing in the latest style. This may involve a skirt or fitted slacks, blouse, jacket, nylons, and attractive shoes. She wears jeans and casual sweaters for relaxation, with comfortable shoes. Tom wants to know if he should bring these types of clothes from home, or if he should go out and buy coordinated sweat suits and sneakers. What would you tell him, and what is the reasoning for your answer?

42. Ingrid is in a grooming group with three other women. She attends well for the first 5 minutes and then starts asking if she can leave. When she is not allowed to leave, she begins to talk to the other women and distracts them. The group is a part of her intervention plan, and she is supposed to attend. How would you deal with Ingrid's behavior?

43. Ingrid's children come to visit her, and she starts crying and asks them to take her out of this prison. How would you respond to this?

44. The children arrive during one of your OT sessions, and she is distracted by their presence. You are working with Ingrid on some simple cognitive activities (games, pegboards). Is there a way that you could incorporate their presence into your intervention session?

45. Ingrid goes out for a day with her husband. They go to lunch and shopping at a department store. When she returns, Tom reports that she was very confused and disoriented. She could not focus on any of the activities, and he had to leave the restaurant before their meal came as Ingrid got quite loud and rude to the staff. He is quite upset about this and is not sure how realistic he has been about her recovery. What do you tell him?

46. Ingrid frequently has angry outbursts when Tom attempts to help her as the rehabilitation team has taught him to. How would you deal with this situation? Are there strategies they could use to minimize these outbursts?

47. Ingrid has progressed to a Level VI on the Rancho Los Amigos Scale in her cognitive function. She requires a wheelchair for mobility when she is fatigued and uses a large base quad cane with supervision at other times. She is going to be discharged home. What safety issues would you want to educate her family about?

Discharge Planning

48. What services would you recommend for Ingrid on her discharge from the rehab hospital if she were at a Rancho Los Amigos Level VI or VII? How would they differ and why?

49. What services would you recommend for Ingrid? Do you think she would benefit more from therapy in outpatient or home care? Why?

50. Write a discharge referral for Ingrid.

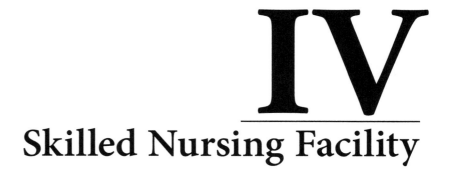

IV
Skilled Nursing Facility

Larry: Chronic Obstructive Pulmonary Disease

Kimberly Witkowski, MS, OTR/L

OCCUPATIONAL PROFILE

Larry is an 82-year-old, right-hand-dominant, Irish American man with a primary diagnosis of chronic obstructive pulmonary disease (COPD) and secondary diagnoses of diabetes and bilateral knee pain. Before his admission, Larry was living at home with his wife, Marie, in a duplex they bought soon after they were married. The bedrooms and full bath are on the second level, and there is a half bath on the first floor, along with the family room and kitchen. Larry and Marie enjoy playing cribbage, watching game shows, and visiting with their grandchildren. They have stopped going out with friends because many of them are experiencing health issues as well. In the past, they also enjoyed going to dances, and Larry participated in the local bowling league for many years before his retirement. He has two grown children—a son who is a successful businessman and lives out of state and a daughter who lives in the other half of their duplex house with her family. Their daughter helps with the vacuuming and grocery shopping and drives her parents to their medical appointments. Marie continues to do the meal preparation, light housekeeping, and laundry.

Larry is a Korean War veteran and served in the U.S. Navy. During his time on active duty, he trained to be a welder and continued to be a professional welder as a civilian. He owned his own company and is still considered an expert in the field by many of his peers. He was forced to retire when he was 64 years old because of his medical conditions. He used to do occasional consults for the welder who took over his business, but these are rare at this time.

Larry has been managing his health care for COPD independently for the past 15 years, including medication and supplemental oxygen at night. About 6 months ago, he started to require more rest breaks and could no longer climb the stairs to enter his home or to his second-floor bedroom. He contracted the flu over the winter and required an acute care hospitalization. He was admitted to long-term care from the hospital because he was not able to walk up the stairs in his home. Larry's goal is to be discharged home, although the team is unsure if this is a safe plan because of his compromised medical status. Larry is being seen in a Veteran's Affairs Facility and has Medicare Part A.

Lowenstein NA, Halloran P.
Case Studies Through the Health Care Continuum:
A Workbook for the Occupational Therapy Student, Second Edition (pp 53-55).
© 2015 SLACK Incorporated.

ANALYSIS OF OCCUPATIONAL PERFORMANCE

Upon admission, Larry was screened by OT and PT, and an OT evaluation was requested to further evaluate his functional status. The Minimum Data Set was completed after Larry's first week in long-term care, and an interdisciplinary team meeting was scheduled to discuss his intervention plan.

The results of Larry's ADLs assessment are as follows: he required use of the hospital bed rail to sit up at the edge of his bed and was able to sit without support at the edge of his bed for approximately 10 minutes before needing a back support. He required maximum assistance to wash and dress his lower body and minimal assistance to wash and dress his upper body. He completed a stand step transfer from his bed to a manual wheelchair with setup and contact guard assistance. He has a rollator walker, but did not use it during transfers. He required close supervision and use of the grab bars to transfer to and from the toilet. He was able to manage his own clothing; however, he had to hold onto the grab bar with one hand while lowering and raising his pants.

Larry's UE AROM is within functional limits, and his manual muscle test resulted in 4/5 bilateral shoulders, with 5/5 in his elbows and wrists. He has fair standing balance and requires use of a rollator for ambulation. He was noted to be short of breath after 1 minute of standing and after 10 minutes of seated ADL. He wore 2 liters of oxygen via nasal canula throughout the evaluation to maintain a blood oxygen saturation above 92%. Sensation was assessed using the Semmes Weinstein (Antibes, France) monofilaments, and he was noted to have diminished light touch in both hands at and distal to the wrist. During this evaluation, Larry was noted to have difficulty remembering the names of the facility, his treating physician, and his OT clinician.

The Allen Cognitive Level Screen (ACLS; Allen et al., 2007) was administered during the second day of evaluation because Larry was unable to tolerate additional testing after ADL and physical assessment. He took 45 minutes and received a score of 5.4 on the ACLS.

QUESTIONS

Occupations

1. What areas of occupation, besides ADLs, would be appropriate to address during Larry's OT interventions?

2. Write out an occupation-based intervention session plan for Larry that could be completed in the OT gym area for one of the occupations identified in Question 1.

3. Would you include meal preparation in your intervention? Why or why not?

Performance Patterns

4. What routines have been affected by Larry's COPD?

5. What roles have been affected by his COPD?

6. If you were using the Model of Human Occupation as your frame of reference, how might you address these during your intervention?

Performance Skills

7. Identify 10 primary performance skills that are affecting Larry's ability to engage in his meaningful occupations.

8. The ACLS is a screening tool for cognition. What information does his current score give you, and how might his ACLS score influence his intervention plan and goals?

9. What other assessments are available to evaluate cognition, and what would your reasoning be to use these versus the ACL battery? Can you identify a functional assessment and a component skills assessment? Which would you prefer to use with Larry and why?

10. How would you explain to Larry the role of OT in rehabilitating his endurance and how it is different from PT?

Client Factors

11. Identify 10 body functions that positively and negatively affect Larry's ability to engage in his daily and meaningful occupations.

12. Give an example of how you would modify an ADLs intervention addressing Larry's endurance or strength to compensate for his cognitive limitations.

13. Larry requires supplemental oxygen via a nasal cannula, with a doctor's order to maintain his oxygen saturation above 92%. When and how would you check this vital sign? What should you include in your documentation?

14. A common intervention for shortness of breath is pursed-lip breathing. How would you teach this technique to Larry? Develop an educational handout of this for him.

15. How was endurance evaluated and measured? What other methods of assessment for endurance would be beneficial to use with Larry?

16. Create an intervention using activity or occupation intervention methods to address Larry's endurance and strength.

Contexts and Environments

17. Identify personal and temporal contexts that would influence your assessment and intervention planning. Explain why you chose these.

18. What social supports are available to Larry and his wife? How might you use these during intervention?

19. How would Larry's home environment influence your intervention planning?

20. Explain to Larry how to use a sock aide. Why would you suggest he use this tool? Does his cognition affect his ability to learn to use adaptive equipment?

21. What additional items of adaptive equipment might be appropriate to try with Larry? Why?

22. In addition to Larry and his family, who else would you educate about Larry's intervention plan?

23. Describe a meeting with Larry's wife and daughter to understand their expectations of Larry upon his return home.

24. What adaptations would you recommend that Larry's wife and daughter complete before he returns home?

Theory and Evidence

25. What theory/theories or frame(s) of reference might you use in developing an intervention plan? Describe the rationale for your choice(s).

26. What, if any, evidence can you find to support your choice of theory/theories and/or frame(s) of reference?

27. What, if any, evidence can you find to support intervention?

Intervention Plan and Goals

28. Prioritize those of Larry's problems that OT would address.

29. Why did you put them in the order you did? Did you consider Larry's goals and priorities?

30. Write a list of long- and short-term goals for Larry's ADL.

31. Are there standardized assessments for ADL that would be appropriate to use during Larry's evaluation? Why or why not?

32. What other assessments might you want to administer and why?

Situations

33. Larry continues to have decreased endurance when walking and will need a wheelchair for functional mobility around the facility and when he is in the community with his family. He is requesting a power wheelchair because he believes he will be too tired from pushing a manual wheelchair. How would you determine if he would benefit from a manual wheelchair vs a power wheelchair? How would you explain your reasoning to Larry and his family? How would you justify a power wheelchair to the VA?

34. Larry arrives to your intervention session without his oxygen and is not sure if he still needs to wear oxygen. What should you do? Give two examples of how you would be able to determine if he needs his oxygen and the reasoning for your primary method to obtain this information.

35. After 1 month of therapy, Larry has made some gains in endurance and ADL, but is not meeting his goals in the set time frames. His insurance company is hesitant to pay for further intervention sessions. Write a sample statement explaining his progress, possible complications with intervention, and your rationale for continued intervention.

Discharge Planning

36. What would you anticipate Larry's functional status to be at discharge from OT services? Check your written goals (Question 30) to ensure that they reflect the expected level of functioning at discharge.

37. You are asked to assist with Larry's discharge planning. What recommendations would you make based on your observations during intervention sessions?

38. In addition to intervention observations, what assessments (standardized or clinical observations) could you use to determine if Larry can safely be discharged to his home?

REFERENCE

Allen, C. K., Austin, S. L., David, S. K., Earhart, C. A., McCraith, D. B., & Riska-Williams, L. (2007). *Allen Cognitive Level Screen—5 (ACLS-5)*. Camarillo, CA: ACLS and LACLS Committee.

Paula: Parkinson's Disease

OCCUPATIONAL PROFILE

Paula is a 76-year-old White woman with a diagnosis of Parkinson's disease and secondary diagnoses of cataracts and hypertension. Paula is retired from her job as a professor of history at an area college. Before her admission to the skilled nursing facility (SNF), Paula was living at home with her husband, Dave, and had been receiving home care services for bathing, dressing, laundry, and light housekeeping 7 days a week. Paula and Dave both receive Meals on Wheels 5 days a week. The home care agency had to cut back on the services they were providing because of changes in Medicare reimbursement, and this left a hole in Paula's ability to remain at home with her elderly husband, who is unable to care for her and the home. She was admitted to the SNF in the town where she and her husband have lived for 45 years.

Although retired as a history professor, Paula kept up with colleagues at the college where she taught, maintained an office at the college (although she rarely went in), and had contact with former students and colleagues by e-mail.

She spent much of her time at the computer in her home office. She continued to review manuscripts for a publishing company as well for as a professional journal.

Paula and Dave have one daughter, but she lives far away and cannot be a part of their daily support services. She is in touch with her parents every few days by phone and visits every other month. Their daughter works and has two small children of her own.

Paula is a strong-willed and independent person who does not like being in the SNF, but is resigned to it. She did explore assisted living facilities, but she and her husband could not afford them. She misses her husband, the contact with her colleagues, and her own home along with the independence it afforded her.

Paula was admitted into the SNF for long-term care. All residents are screened at admission by OT and PT. Minimum data sets are completed, with each team member completing the appropriate section, and a team meeting is set within 7 days to discuss the intervention plan and goals. Paula's goals are to be able to interact with her colleagues again, to access the community, and keep her relationship with her husband.

Lowenstein NA, Halloran P.
Case Studies Through the Health Care Continuum:
A Workbook for the Occupational Therapy Student, Second Edition (pp 57-60).
© 2015 SLACK Incorporated.

Paula was screened by OT, and a subsequent OT evaluation was requested to gather more data on her functional skills in bathing, dressing, feeding, cognition, and psychosocial status. Paula has Medicare Part A and B. She will not be returning home.

ANALYSIS OF OCCUPATIONAL PERFORMANCE

OT evaluation was completed using chart review, interview, the Canadian Occupational Performance Measure (COPM; Law et al., 1990), observation of functional activities, and motor assessment. With observation, Paula demonstrates intact cognition, sensation, perception, and hearing, but has decreased visual acuity due to cataracts. Her bilateral UE AROM is within functional limits in all movements. Her muscle strength is 4/5 in the shoulder muscles on both sides, and 4+/5 throughout the remainder of her UEs, with her right side being her dominant side. However, she demonstrates poor trunk control and cannot sit unsupported for more than 5 minutes before she begins to slide down and lean to the left in the chair. Paula demonstrates the ability to sit unsupported for about 30 seconds before slouching and lateral trunk flexion to the left begins. Her head is laterally flexed to the left as well. She has decreased neck ROM (both passive and active), with only about a third of full head rotation present. She has decreased gross and fine motor coordination in both UEs. Her handwriting is illegible, and her movements are slow. There are intention tremors in both her UEs, but the tremors increase with effortful activity and make it difficult for her to use her right arm during functional activities. She has tone of 2 on the Ashworth Scale in her LEs, with the left leg having increased tremor and spasticity with effortful movement and at rest. This leg flexes at the knee and hip during any activity in sitting, leading to poor sitting balance. The right leg has mildly increased tremors, but they do not interfere with function. Paula's trunk is rigid and moves as if a log, with no dissociation between her upper and lower trunk.

Paula ambulates with a rolling walker, although she does not like to use it, and ambulates by holding onto the furniture to get to the bed or chair. At home, she experienced frequent falls and had taken to wearing kneepads to protect herself from the inevitable falls. When moved from stand to sit, she gets near the chair or bed and just flops down any old way, sometimes coming close to missing altogether. Bed mobility is independent, but effortful. She is able to roll side to side using the bedrails; she uses the controls of the hospital bed to raise the head of the bed to assist in sitting up.

Paula has difficulty bathing at the sink. She sits on the toilet to sponge bathe her upper body; however, due to her poor sitting balance, she slides off the toilet onto the floor. She is unable to bend over and wash her lower torso and dresses her upper body slowly, while sitting in a supportive chair. Paula requires maximum assistance with dressing her lower body. She has difficulty with buttons, but can eventually get them done. She is dependent for her shoes and socks. She is able to feed herself, but her hands shake when lifting glasses, mugs, and silverware. It takes her a long time to cut up her food and to eat. Her swallowing is intact, but drooling does occur during activities that require a lot of effort.

Paula is short-tempered with the staff, although this is not her usual personality. She states she does not want to participate in the activity program and says the groups are "boring" and for the "mentally challenged." She does not understand what OT is and states she "already has an occupation." She misses her husband, who is still living in their home, and the contact with her academic colleagues and students.

She wants more than anything to be able to bring her computer in and have Internet access so she can stay "mentally with it." She shares a room with another resident who loves to watch TV most of the day. Her roommate leaves the TV on even when she is not there and does not want anyone to turn it off. On the COPM, Paula identified using her computer, communicating with colleagues and her husband, and independence in daily bathing and dressing as her priorities for OT intervention.

QUESTIONS

Occupations

1. What would you identify as major occupations affected by Paula's admission to the SNF? Is it appropriate for OT to address all of these?

2. Given that Medicare is the payer for Paula's OT, how could you address the occupation of communication management, volunteer participation, and social participation with friends outside the SNF?

Performance Patterns

3. How has Paula's admission to the SNF interrupted her roles and routines? Which ones have been most affected?

4. How can OT address this area?

Performance Skills

5. Identify 10 performance skills that are primary obstacles for Paula in being independent in bathing, dressing, and feeding.

6. Identify 10 performance skills that are supports to her engagement in occupations.

7. How would you address Paula's difficulty at mealtime?

8. How would you educate other staff about your mealtime recommendations?

Client Factors

9. Describe Paula's UE deficits. How do these affect her ability to complete her meaningful occupations? Do you feel that addressing these issues would result in her being able to reach her goals? Why or why not?

10. What type of intervention methods would you use to address Paula's musculoskeletal status?

11. How would these methods be differentiated from PT intervention?

12. Parkinson's disease is characterized by rigidity and tremors. How would you address these as they are seen in Paula?

13. Would an exercise program be beneficial for Paula? Please explain your answer.

14. What are the psychosocial issues that you might address with Paula? How would you address these issues in your intervention sessions?

15. What types of groups might be meaningful to Paula? How would you introduce her to these groups so that she would try them? Is it important for Paula to go to groups if she does not want to? Why or why not?

Contexts and Environment

16. Identify personal and temporal factors that could influence your assessment and intervention planning.

17. How might you intervene in the virtual context?

18. What other individuals might you enlist to help Paula's adjustment to the SNF?

19. What type of adaptive equipment would you use with Paula to assist with bathing, dressing, and feeding?

20. How would you teach Paula to use the adaptive equipment recommended?

21. What type of seating equipment would you use to position Paula properly? Remember that customized wheelchairs are not usually paid for when in an SNF.

22. What are some of the safety concerns for Paula? How would you prioritize these?

23. Besides Paula's Parkinson's disease, which other diagnoses could pose safety issues for her and why? How would you go about working with Paula on these issues?

Theory and Evidence

24. What theory/theories or frame(s) of reference might you use in developing an intervention plan? Describe the rationale for your choice(s).

25. What evidence can you find that supports OT intervention for individuals with Parkinson's disease? Would this change your intervention in any way?

26. What evidence can you find to support intervention for tremors?

Intervention Plan and Goals

27. Paula does not have a clear understanding of the role of OT. How would you explain your role to her so that she would be invested in her OT program?

28. Write a problem list for Paula and prioritize the problems according to what you feel would have the most impact on Paula's function and mental health. Explain your reasoning.

29. Write a list of long- and short-term goals for Paula.

30. What part of the assessment and intervention is appropriate for a certified OT assistant to carry out? Why?

31. With which other team members would you consult and collaborate?

Situations

32. At the team meeting, the dietician identifies Paula as a high risk for aspiration and wants to start her on a ground diet. You feel that Paula needs dysphagia intervention before changing her diet. How would you address this issue in the team meeting?

33. The certified nursing assistants see Paula as a difficult resident. She requires a lot of their time at meals and for ADLs because she is so slow. They want to do everything for her so they can get on to their next resident, but Paula gets angry at them because she wants to remain as independent as possible and do as much for herself as she is able. How would you address this issue with the certified nursing assistants who care for Paula daily?

Discharge Planning

34. Paula has refused to participate in intervention for the past week, stating that she just does not feel like doing anything. What are some of the possible reasons for this, and what would you do?

35. How would you ensure that gains made during your OT interventions are maintained once Paula is discharged from therapy?

REFERENCE

Law, M., Baptiste, S., Carswell, A., McColl, M. A., Polatajko, H., & Pollock, N. (1990). *Canadian Occupational Performance Measure.* Ottawa, Canada: Canadian Occupational Therapy Association.

14

Quinn: Dementia

OCCUPATIONAL PROFILE

Quinn is an 87-year-old White man with a diagnosis of dementia. Quinn has a past medical history of congestive heart failure, hypertension, depression, and gout. Quinn has been a resident at the nursing home for the past 2 years. He resides on the long-term care wing of the facility. It is the family's plan that Quinn remain at the nursing home indefinitely.

Quinn's wife, Dorothea, visits on Wednesdays and Fridays. She takes Quinn outside onto the patio and reads him letters from their grandchildren. When she has no family news, she reads him the newspaper or the church bulletin. Dorothea wants Quinn to remain as mentally capable as possible. It is obvious that there is a strong bond between them. Dorothea holds Quinn's hand for her entire visit. She attends all of his care plan meetings and frequently speaks as an advocate on his behalf. They have two children and five grandchildren. They all live within 2 hours of Dorothea and Quinn. They try to visit monthly, but often miss a visit because they have busy lives.

Quinn participates minimally in the facility's activities. If someone wheels him into the day room, he will listen to the radio or watch the entertainers. Quinn speaks only if spoken to or if he needs something. He uses simple sentences and often answers incorrectly when asked simple questions. Quinn recognizes Dorothea, but sometimes confuses his daughters and grandchildren. He cannot recall the names of staff members, but does smile when he sees someone he recognizes.

The nurse, who realized Quinn is now requiring more assistance from the nursing assistants at meals, has referred him to OT for a feeding evaluation. Quinn had been eating in the main dining room for lunch and dinner, but now has to eat in the day room on the unit because he requires assistance with his meals. Such one-on-one assistance is not available in the main dining room.

The nurse and Quinn's primary nursing assistant make it clear that Quinn has been requiring more help with his meals over the past 3 to 4 weeks. In the past, he had required only setup with his meals. Reportedly, he now needs to be fed. Quinn has been dependent for his ADLs since he arrived at the facility and is nonambulatory. The facility staff feels that Quinn is more cognitively impaired than he appears. Quinn is unable to state his goals for OT. He does not appear to understand the purpose of OT. The purpose and projected outcome of OT is explained to his

Lowenstein NA, Halloran P.
Case Studies Through the Health Care Continuum:
A Workbook for the Occupational Therapy Student, Second Edition (pp 61-64).
© 2015 SLACK Incorporated.

wife. She repeats her own goal of having her husband be able to eat in the dining room at meals. She agrees for OT services to begin. Because Quinn is not newly admitted to the facility, it is the policy of the OT department to use a specialized feeding evaluation for long-term residents. He has both Medicare Part A and Medicaid.

ANALYSIS OF OCCUPATIONAL PERFORMANCE

Quinn is evaluated by chart review, interview of the nursing staff, and certified nursing assistants, as well as observation at mealtime and a motor assessment. Quinn is sitting in a manual wheelchair that his family purchased for him several years ago. It has elevating leg rests to prevent LE edema and a reclining back. He is sitting on a combination gel/foam cushion. His seated position on evaluation is as follows: the back is reclined at approximately a 35-degree angle. His pelvis is tilted posteriorly, his head is jutting forward, and his cervical spine is in a kyphotic posture. His feet do not sit flat on the foot pedals when they are in the down position; when the leg rests are elevated, his knees are bent approximately 20 degrees.

Quinn has AROM within normal limits for his UEs with slightly less flexion of the shoulders secondary to the kyphosis. His strength is 4–/5, and his gross motor control is within functional limits. His fine motor coordination is impaired, but could not be formally assessed because of his cognitive status. His sensation appears intact for both UEs, but also could not be formally assessed. He is right-hand dominant.

Cognitively, Quinn displays short- and long-term memory deficits and a decrease in executive functions. He is able to follow simple one-step verbal instructions accompanied by visual cues, such as "shake my hand." He is unable to learn new information, but performs automatic responses without prompting. He has an attention span of approximately 5 minutes. He is oriented to self and his wife. Quinn is on a regular diet.

Quinn requires setup for his meal. He is unable to identify and locate the various utensils used during his meal. However, he is able to demonstrate holding a spoon and a fork correctly once it is placed in his hand. Quinn has difficulty scooping the food onto the spoon. He is unable to successfully pierce food with a fork on 6 out of 10 tries. Quinn frequently drops the food once he has successfully gotten it onto his utensil. While bringing it to his mouth, many pieces fall into his lap. Quinn then puts the fork or spoon down and picks the pieces up with his fingers; he gets the pieces of food into his mouth every time.

Quinn is able to eat a piece of buttered bread independently once it is placed in his hand. Quinn is also able to hold a cup independently, but, again, only after it is placed in his hand. He is only able to drink half of his liquid because he cannot extend his neck from the flexed position to tip the remainder of the liquid out of the glass. He is able to continue drinking once given a straw. However, he neglects to use the straw the next time the cup is placed in his hand. Quinn does not finish his drink without assistance. He uses his napkin spontaneously once it is placed in his hand.

QUESTIONS

Occupations

1. Although feeding is the occupation that Quinn was referred for, do you think working on this skill might translate into other occupations? If so, which ones and why?

2. Describe a single OT intervention session with Quinn, focusing on increasing independence at meals.

Performance Patterns

3. How might his wife's roles and routines affect your intervention? Would you include her in any of your intervention sessions?

4. What impact do you think Quinn's inability to feed himself may have on his wife?

Performance Skills

5. Identify 10 key performance skills that have a negative impact on Quinn's ability to self-feed.

6. Identify 10 performance skills that are strengths for his ability to self-feed.

7. What techniques might you use to facilitate the skills needed to improve his self-feeding abilities?

8. Using Figure 14-1, describe what is correct and incorrect with Quinn's wheelchair positioning.

9. You adjust Quinn's wheelchair so he sits upright at a 90-degree angle. He slowly begins to slip out of his chair. Explain what you would do in this situation.

10. How would you modify Quinn's wheelchair to produce a better seated position?

11. Make a list of all the possible complications Quinn might have because of his position in the wheelchair.

Client Factors

12. Identify 10 body functions that have the greatest impact on Quinn's feeding skills.

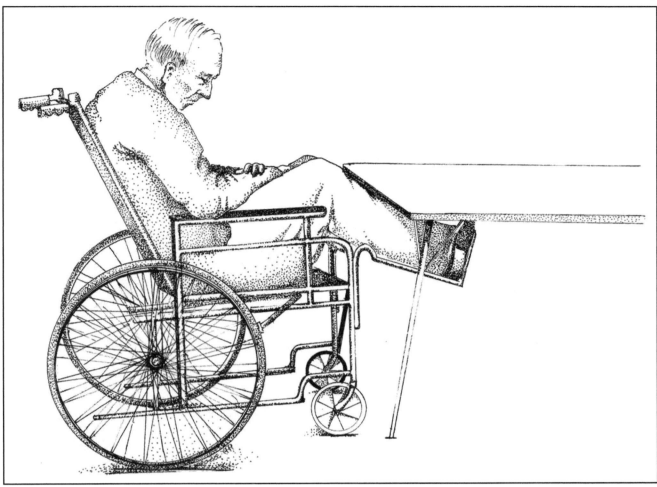

Figure 14-1. Quinn's wheelchair positioning.

13. What can be done to improve Quinn's fine motor coordination?

14. What strategies would you use for his cognitive deficits during feeding?

Contexts and Environment

15. What type of environmental adaptations should be made to allow Quinn to feed himself more independently?

16. What type of adaptive equipment might Quinn need to enable him to be independent in self-feeding? Would you recommend adaptive equipment for someone with Alzheimer's disease? Why or why not?

17. How does food texture influence self-feeding? Do you think Quinn needs a change of texture?

18. Explain how you would involve the dietary and nursing staff in your intervention.

19. What type of support do you think might benefit Dorothea as Quinn's condition progresses? To which other disciplines might you refer Dorothea? Identify resources in your community to support Dorothea.

Theory and Evidence

20. What theory/theories or frame(s) of reference might you use in developing an intervention plan? Describe the rationale for your choice(s).

21. What, if any, evidence can you find to support your choice of theory/theories and/or frame(s) of reference?

22. Is there evidence to support feeding intervention for individuals with dementia?

Intervention Plan and Goals

23. Identify the key issues affecting Quinn's ability to feed himself.

24. Write out a problem list.

25. Identify standardized assessments that would assist your intervention planning in this situation.

26. What short-term goals would you set for Quinn to help reach the long-term goal of eating in the main dining room?

27. What are strengths that could help Quinn achieve his wife's and the staff's goals?

28. What are deficits that may impede achievement of identified goals?

29. Write a specific intervention plan for Quinn, including frequency and duration.

30. Who might be a primary payer for these services? How would you justify payment?

Situations

31. You have made changes in Quinn's mealtime routine and want other staff members to follow through with your interventions. Name all the staff positions that would be involved and what instructions you would give them to ensure the desired program carryover occurs.

32. Quinn becomes agitated when you try to rearrange his plate to facilitate independence. He refuses to eat after you have intervened. What would you do?

33. Dorothea decides to visit Quinn during the day at lunch. She wants him to sit on the patio with her. There is no table out there. What adaptations would you need to make to enable Quinn to eat his lunch on the patio with Dorothea?

34. You arrive at the facility early and go in to see how Quinn is doing with his breakfast. You see his nursing assistant feeding him oatmeal. What do you do?

35. This same scenario occurs several days in a row. What might be some of the reasons as to why the nursing assistants keep feeding him day after day?

36. How would you deal with staff members enabling Quinn's dependence at meals?

Discharge Planning

37. When you decide to discharge Quinn from OT services, what would you need to have in place to ensure he is able to maintain his current level of independence?

38. How could you monitor Quinn to see that he does not return to being fed at meals?

V

Outpatient Rehabilitation

Ursula: Right Carpal Tunnel Repair, Left Carpal Tunnel Syndrome

OCCUPATIONAL PROFILE

Ursula is a 34-year-old, married Black female. She works as a hairdresser in a busy salon in an urban area. Ursula and her husband have four children between the ages of 7 and 15 years. Her husband works as a factory foreman. She needs to maintain a certain number of clients each month to make it worth the money she pays the salon owner for the rental of the chair. This requires that she work 6 days a week. She takes only a lunch break and a short cigarette break in the morning and afternoon each day. Ursula can make her own hours, but she has to let the receptionist know what hours she will be working each week.

Ursula and her husband share the responsibilities of the household, including the cooking, grocery shopping, and duties of getting the children where they have to go. Although their schedules do not allow a lot of time together, Ursula and her husband are very close and make sure that Sunday is a family day.

Ursula is a deeply religious woman. She enjoys her work as a hairdresser, and she is also an active church volunteer. Her children all are active in the church youth group as well. Ursula and her husband enjoy bowling and, in the winter, try to bowl one night a week.

Ursula is an energetic woman with an upbeat disposition and outlook on life. She came from a large southern family and was one of the youngest. There is not much that bothers her. She states she gets her strength from her church and family.

Ursula's symptoms have been apparent for the past 6 months. Initially, she noticed that, by her lunch break, she had a tingling in her right hand. This usually went away by the time lunch was over. After a few weeks, she became aware that, by evening, her right hand was tingling and felt like it had "fallen asleep." She started to drop silverware when trying to prepare dinner. By bedtime, her right arm would be feeling tired and painful. At first, the symptoms disappeared by morning, but soon she noticed that her right hand and arm hurt all the time—at some times more than at others. On a few occasions, she almost dropped the hair dryer when she was drying a client's hair. After this had happened a few times, she decided to see her primary care physician, who suggested she wear a wrist support that she could buy at the local pharmacy. This helped for a short time, but the symptoms never completely went away.

Lowenstein NA, Halloran P.
Case Studies Through the Health Care Continuum:
A Workbook for the Occupational Therapy Student, Second Edition (pp 67-70).
© 2015 SLACK Incorporated.

Ursula was then referred to a hand specialist who tried anti-inflammatory medications, injections, a custom-made splint, and rest for 1 week. This also helped, but, as soon as she returned to work, the symptoms returned. Ursula did not wear the splint at work because it hindered her use of the scissors and hair dryer. The hand specialist diagnosed her with carpal tunnel syndrome and recommended surgery to release the nerve compression and alleviate the symptoms. In the meantime, Ursula also had symptoms of carpal tunnel syndrome in her left hand, but the physician felt that, because this was in the early stages, it could be treated more conservatively. Ursula's goals are to return to work at her previous level in 2 weeks. She says that if she does not pay the rent on the chair, the salon owner will just rent it to someone else; many hairdressers want to work in this salon.

ANALYSIS OF OCCUPATIONAL PERFORMANCE

Ursula was evaluated by OT in the outpatient clinic 2 weeks post-surgery for rehabilitation of the right hand and to address the deteriorating function of the left hand. She has sensory deficits for light touch, deep pressure, hot–cold, and sharp–dull along the median nerve distribution of both hands, with the right hand being worse than the left. Ursula is right-handed. Formal testing using the Moberg pickup test (Moberg, 1958) and the Jebsen Hand Function Test (Jebsen, Taylor, Treischmann, Trotter, & Howard, 1969) showed a significant decrease in fine motor coordination. Strength was tested on the left hand with a dynamometer and registered 25 pounds. The right hand was not tested because of the recent surgery. Her AROM in both UEs is within functional limits. However, the strength in her right shoulder is 3+/5. Her left shoulder is 4/5. Both elbows are 4/5. Ursula reports some pain at the right wrist where the surgery was performed, but it occurs mostly with activity. Her left wrist and hand continue to have paresthesia upon wrist flexion. Both hands have decreased pinch strength for two-point, three-point, and lateral pinches. Ursula has slight edema of the right hand and fingers.

Ursula is independent in functional mobility and all transfers. She has difficulty with ADLs, especially tasks that require fine motor skills. Ursula's husband or oldest daughter have been helping her get dressed since the surgery. She needs help with her bra, shoe laces, buttons, zippers, and socks. She has difficulty washing, but will not let anyone help her. Meal preparation is difficult, and her husband has been doing it since her surgery. He is also doing the housework, and Ursula feels bad about her inability to help with the home management tasks.

She is anxious to get better and says she will comply with any program she is given. Her family is very supportive.

Ursula's goals are to get back to the salon in 2 weeks; to be able to dress, shower, and wash herself; and to be pain free and able to care for her family and her home.

QUESTIONS

Occupation

1. Identify the occupations in which Ursula is having difficulty engaging.

2. Identify the occupations in which Ursula is able to engage well.

3. How would you address Ursula's dressing deficits while working in an outpatient department?

4. What home management tasks will be difficult for Ursula to do for the next month?

5. What home management tasks will Ursula be able to do within 2 weeks, and will these tasks need modifications? If so, what should these modifications be?

6. Ursula talked about her leisure interests during the initial evaluation. What are they, and how will her carpal tunnel syndrome affect her ability to pursue them?

Performance Patterns

7. What roles have been affected by Ursula's carpal tunnel in her UEs? Do you feel she will be able to successfully resume all these roles? How long might you expect her recovery to take?

8. What routines have been disrupted by Ursula's carpal tunnel syndrome? Has she managed to adapt any of these routines? How might you assist her in adapting one of these routines?

Performance Skills

9. Identify 10 key performance skills that have been affected negatively by Ursula's carpal tunnel syndrome and her surgery.

10. Identify 10 key performance skills that have not been affected and can be considered strengths in developing an intervention plan.

11. Do an activity analysis of Ursula's job as a hairdresser.

12. What level of hand function does Ursula need to return to her job?

Client Factors

13. What is the importance of Ursula's spirituality for your OT intervention?

14. What values and beliefs are important to keep in mind when developing your goals? Why?

15. Identify 10 key body functions that have been negatively affected by Ursula's carpal tunnel syndrome and her surgery.

16. Identify 10 key body functions that are strengths that will assist Ursula's recovery.

17. Which nerve is involved with carpal tunnel syndrome? What are the motor and sensory distributions of this nerve?

18. Write a protocol for Ursula to follow to control the edema in her fingers.

19. Write a home exercise program for Ursula to follow for weeks 1 and 2 of outpatient therapy. What type of exercises would you prescribe and why? Can you think of a way of embedding these exercises into daily tasks? If so, describe a few.

20. Ursula has the beginnings of carpal tunnel syndrome in her left hand, and her doctor wishes to treat it without surgery. What interventions would you use for her left hand?

21. What is the purpose of wearing a splint for carpal tunnel syndrome?

22. What type of splint, if any, would you make for Ursula, and what material would you use? Please write out a wearing schedule for the splint for week 1. How would this differ from week 2 and beyond?

23. Ursula has some significant sensory deficits in her right hand. How would you address these in your intervention sessions? Would you suggest any home activities for her and, if so, what would they be? What impact might these sensory issues have on her work as a hairdresser?

24. While doing some gross motor coordination activities, you notice that Ursula is able to reach the object, but she is moving her whole body, and her shoulder is elevated and abducted when she attempts to reach. What is the most likely cause of this, and what would you do to address this?

25. What types of hand and wrist movements should someone who has carpal tunnel syndrome avoid making?

Contexts and Environment

26. Identify personal and temporal factors that may influence your assessment and intervention planning.

27. Identify cultural factors that may influence your assessment and intervention planning.

28. What, if any, adaptive equipment would Ursula benefit from for self-care tasks? What is the cost of this equipment?

29. What, if any, adaptive equipment would Ursula benefit from for meal preparation? What is the cost of this equipment?

30. Ursula's carpal tunnel syndrome occurred because of her job. What, if any, modifications or adaptations would you suggest she adopt at work? Why?

31. Can you find ergonomic tools in a catalogue or store for Ursula to start using? What do they cost? If you cannot find any, how might you adapt those tools she already has to prevent further cumulative trauma disorder?

32. What adaptations would you suggest Ursula make in her daily routine as it applies to her job?

Theory and Evidence

33. What theory/theories or frame(s) of reference might you use in developing an intervention plan? Describe the rationale for your choice(s).

34. What, if any, evidence can you find to support your choice of theory/theories and/or frame(s) of reference?

35. What evidence can you find to develop an intervention for carpal tunnel syndrome? Does this use occupation, activity, or preparatory methods?

36. If the evidence uses preparatory methods or tasks, how could you adapt this so that you use occupations or activities as intervention methods?

Intervention Plan and Goals

37. What are your long- and short-term goals for Ursula?

38. What is the first priority to address and why?

39. For which aspects of Ursula's intervention could COTA be responsible?

40. What, if any, obstacles do you see to Ursula's recovery? How might you address these?

41. What is the role of physical agent modalities in OT? Can COTAs use them? Who is responsible for establishing competency for the use of these modalities?

42. What, if any, physical agent modalities would you use during Ursula's OT sessions? Why would you use these modalities, and how would you address their use in relation to purposeful activity?

Situations

43. Ursula is having a difficult time coping with her recovery. She feels it is going too slowly and that the doctor lied to her about how fast it would take her to recover. She is getting discouraged and saying things like, "I'll have to give up my chair at the salon." She has also noted that she is doing her home exercise program only when she feels like it, "since it doesn't seem to be helping any." How would you address her psychological state?

44. Ursula usually comes to therapy alone, but one day her husband accompanies her to see how her therapy is going. It is a typical busy day, and you are seeing two patients at a time. While one is doing an activity, you are working with the other. The patients are close enough so that, after the session, Ursula's husband pulls you aside and angrily accuses you of spending more time with the other patient than with Ursula and says you did that because the other patient is "richer" than Ursula. How would you handle this situation?

Discharge Planning

45. Ursula does not understand what carpal tunnel syndrome is or why she has it. Create a patient information booklet for her and her family.

46. Ursula is to be discharged from outpatient therapy after 4 weeks. She has made gains in all areas of range of movement, strength grasp, and pinch strength, but these have not returned to what they should be for her age and profession. Her sensory deficits, although still present, do not bother her much. She can dress herself, but her hands are still fatigued by the end of the day. What type of home program would you send home with Ursula, and how would you impress upon her the importance of following it?

47. Write a discharge note to Ursula's hand surgeon.

REFERENCES

Jebsen, R. H., Taylor, N., Treischmann, R. B., Trotter, M. J., & Howard, L. A. (1969). An objective and standardized test of hand function. *Archives of Physical Medicine and Rehabilitation, 50,* 311–319.

Moberg, E. (1958). Objective methods for determining the functional value of sensibility in the hand. *Journal of Bone and Joint Surgery British, 40B,* 454–476.

16

Xavier: Bilateral Elbow Tendonitis

OCCUPATIONAL PROFILE

Xavier is a 33-year-old Latino man. His primary language is Spanish and, although he does understand English, his own oral communication in English is problematic. He does not read English. He has a diagnosis of bilateral tendonitis, or, more specifically, lateral epicondylitis. He has no other significant medical history or problems. His primary physician referred him for outpatient OT. Xavier reportedly has been experiencing worsening pain over the past 4 months. He works as a printer for a large commercial printing company. He is married, has twin 8-year-old boys, and his wife is expecting their third child. She also speaks Spanish as her home language and has difficulty with English. Their sons are fluent in both English and Spanish. Xavier is angry about the onset of the tendonitis and is clearly frustrated that his pain is slowing him down. Xavier prides himself on being a good worker.

Xavier is experiencing no functional limitations at home as a result of the tendonitis, but is worried about how much longer he is going to be able to perform at his current job. Xavier has given up his favorite activity, working out at the gym, because of his elbow pain. He says he uses ice on his elbows at night, which seems to help "un poco" (a little).

Through a medical interpreter, it was learned that Xavier has been a printer for 13 years. He took a new job running a large press almost 1 year ago. He says that, when he first began, he noticed the discomfort in his elbows. After a year of working, frequent trips to the gym, and taking vitamins, Xavier reports the pain to be increasingly worse. He operates a 40-inch press. He says that loading the paper into the press causes him the most pain. He describes having to lift 40-inch wide paper off skids from the floor onto a platform on the press. He lifts the paper in increments of approximately 30 pounds at a time, up to 3,000 to 4,000 pounds a day. He also has to fan the paper out to allow air in between the sheets before it is printed on. Xavier explains this step as essential because, without it, the paper will stick together and the press will jam. The motion of fanning the paper starts in pronation and moves through supination to the end range.

Xavier says he first started with pain much worse in the right arm; now his left arm feels just as bad. He says that sometimes, after a particularly busy workday, he is awakened at night from the pain. Xavier remarks that it is inconsistent, however, and the pain occasionally wakes him up at night during weekends as well.

Lowenstein NA, Halloran P.
Case Studies Through the Health Care Continuum:
A Workbook for the Occupational Therapy Student, Second Edition (pp 71-73).
© 2015 SLACK Incorporated.

Xavier is responsible for all home repair, car maintenance, and yard work at home. He and his family live in a small home. His wife works as well and is responsible for all the housekeeping and child care. Xavier reports pain at times when playing ball with his sons.

ANALYSIS OF OCCUPATIONAL PERFORMANCE

Xavier was seen for an OT evaluation. He has no cognitive, perceptual, visual, hearing, or sensory deficits. A medical interpreter was used during the evaluation. He has AROM in normal ranges for bilateral UEs, although he reports pain during wrist extension and supination. Despite the pain, his strength is also normal. Xavier is right-handed and has no coordination deficits, edema, or skin changes.

Xavier is independent in all self-care and work tasks. He has lost no time from his work because of the tendonitis, although he reports wanting to leave early many days because of the pain. He continues driving and had not experienced inability in doing any of his normal daily tasks. Xavier's goal from therapy is to be pain-free. He agrees to participate in OT and remarks, "I'm tired of dealing with this pain."

QUESTIONS

Occupations

1. Which occupation(s) are most affected by Xavier's diagnosis?

2. Which occupation(s) would you suggest Xavier not participate in while he is receiving OT?

3. Xavier would like to continue his workouts at the gym 3 days per week. What would you suggest?

Performance Patterns

4. What roles have been most affected by Xavier's diagnosis and pain?

5. What routines would you want to find out more about? Why?

6. Identify areas for client education. How would you write a handout for Xavier on one of these areas?

7. Why is it important to educate Xavier regarding his part in the intervention program?

Performance Skills

8. Identify 10 performance skills that would have a negative impact on Xavier's ability to participate in his meaningful occupations.

9. Identify 10 performance skills that would have a positive impact on your OT intervention.

10. Describe an intervention session that uses meaningful activities as your primary intervention method. What equipment or tools would you need to complete this activity?

Client Factors

11. What values do you feel will be helpful to Xavier's engagement in OT? Why?

12. Identify 10 body structures that may be affecting Xavier's ability to engage in meaningful occupations.

13. What types of physical agent modalities would you use for Xavier's tendonitis? Explain why and who is qualified to administer them.

14. Write out a home program for Xavier to follow. Be sure to include all information needed for a thorough, effective home program. How would you complete this task, given that Xavier does not read English?

15. Why do you think Xavier is angry about having tendonitis?

16. Why is it so important psychologically for Xavier to have this intervention be successful?

17. If Xavier's tendonitis continued, what kind of effect would it have on him?

Contexts and Environment

18. What cultural considerations would you want to take into account when working with Xavier? How would you do this?

19. Identify personal and temporal factors that could influence your assessment and intervention planning.

20. What adaptations could be made to Xavier's workstation that would be less likely to exacerbate the tendonitis?

21. What actions should Xavier take to lessen his pain?

22. What precautions should Xavier take to prevent worsening his tendonitis?

23. What social supports do you think you could call on for Xavier?

Theory and Evidence

24. What theory/theories or frame(s) of reference might you use in developing an intervention plan? Describe the rationale for your choice(s).

25. What, if any, evidence can you find to support your choice of theory/theories and/or frame(s) of reference?

26. What, if any, evidence can you find to support intervention?

Intervention Plan and Goals

27. What would you and Xavier set as his short-term goals? His long-term goals?

28. Write an intervention plan for Xavier, including frequency and duration.

29. What evidence can you find to support intervention for Xavier's diagnosis?

30. What theoretical model would you use to guide your intervention?

Situations

31. Xavier attends OT, but there is no interpreter available. He has brought his sons with him because his wife is working and they cannot be left alone. What would you do?

32. Xavier is making good progress and reporting less pain after 1 week of intervention. His insurance company wants to limit him to only one more visit. Explain what you would do.

33. The insurance company case manager tells you she thought Xavier was going to be having PT rather than OT and wants him to change to PT. What would you say and do?

34. You suspect that Xavier is not following his home program because he cannot demonstrate his exercises when you ask him to. Identify some reasons you think this might be, as well as some solutions.

35. Xavier tells you he has been trying to keep his tendonitis a secret from his employers. He asks you if you think this is a good idea. What is your response? Why?

Discharge Planning

36. How long would you anticipate seeing Xavier for OT intervention if he continues with his current job?

37. If Xavier reported his pain to be present, but less pronounced, what would you recommend that he do to meet his goals of being pain-free?

Yolanda: Left Fractured Humerus

OCCUPATIONAL PROFILE

Yolanda is a 45-year-old female who identifies as Black. She fell and sustained a proximal oblique fracture of the shaft of her left humerus while bird watching. Additional diagnoses include diverticulitis, osteoporosis, and alcohol abuse. Yolanda is an avid birdwatcher and goes out with friends to different areas several mornings a week She was walking along a wooded path looking through her binoculars when she tripped and fell over a log. She put out her left arm to stop the fall (the right was holding the binoculars) and heard a crack as soon as she landed. The pain was excruciating, and her friends immediately took her to the nearest emergency department. X-rays showed a fracture of the upper humerus. Her arm was placed in a sling, and no surgery was required, but the fracture is too high to immobilize with a cast.

Before her accident, Yolanda had no deficits in her daily life. She drove, cooked, shopped, and took care of the family finances. She has been married to her second husband for 15 years and has two teenage children from her first marriage. She and her husband, Bob, enjoy traveling and entertaining. She lives in a large, two-story suburban home and does not work. Her husband is an investment banker, and they are well-off financially. He often works late, coming home around 9 p.m. most weeknights. Yolanda's children are very active in their after-school activities, and Yolanda likes to volunteer to help with these activities as needed.

Yolanda has a history of alcohol abuse, but claims she has stopped drinking. She is a personable woman, but is very private and does not like to talk about herself or her family. She has always felt that she is an independent woman, who enjoys the company of others, especially women, but does not want to rely on anyone except her husband. She says her goals are to return to her previous activity level and occupations.

Yolanda is 6 weeks post-fracture and will be seen in the outpatient clinic for OT to address the fractured humerus, with discharge to her own care when therapy is complete. Her insurance company has approved an initial eight visits, including evaluation.

Lowenstein NA, Halloran P.
Case Studies Through the Health Care Continuum:
A Workbook for the Occupational Therapy Student, Second Edition (pp 75-77).
© 2015 SLACK Incorporated.

ANALYSIS OF OCCUPATIONAL PERFORMANCE

Yolanda was evaluated through chart review, interview, and motor assessment. She does not appear to have any perceptual, visual, or hearing deficits, although she wears glasses for reading. Sensation is intact, although she complains of occasional tingling in her left hand. She appears somewhat forgetful during the evaluation, and it is difficult to get a good history of events from her.

Yolanda is right-handed and expresses relief that it is her left arm that is broken rather than the right. Strength cannot be assessed because of non–weight-bearing precautions. Yolanda has pain with movement of the shoulder in flexion beyond 25 degrees and extension beyond 10 degrees. Her arm will be immobilized in a sling for at least two more weeks, except for when she is showering, dressing, or in therapy. She has AROM in her elbow 0 to 110 before pain; wrist and fingers are within normal limits. Coordination is impaired because of immobilization. Her right arm shows no deficits in strength, AROM, or coordination. Yolanda has difficulty getting up from low furniture, but has found that if she sits in a chair with arms, she can get up more easily. She has difficulty in general with going from sit to stand or supine to stand because of her inability to use her left arm to assist. She requires assistance with dressing and fasteners. She has figured out how to brush her teeth and comb her hair but cannot pull it back, which is how she normally wears it. She has permission to shower, but has been too fearful to try it. She is dependent for all meal preparation, so her family often gets takeout meals or else goes out to eat after the girls' school activities.

Yolanda considers her fracture to be a stupid accident and a great inconvenience. She and her husband have a 4-week trip coming up in 3 weeks, and she does not want to be hampered with a sling and pain. She would like to be able to go on her trip without the sling. Her doctor's orders are for pendulum exercises, active assistive, and active exercises as tolerated.

QUESTIONS

Occupations

1. Identify the ADL occupations most affected by Yolanda's injury.

2. Identify the IADL occupations most affected by Yolanda's injury.

3. Identify the rest and sleep occupations most affected by Yolanda's injury.

4. Identify the work occupations most affected by Yolanda's injury.

5. Identify the leisure occupations most affected by Yolanda's injury.

6. Identify the social participation occupations most affected by Yolanda's injury.

7. Prioritize these occupations for your outpatient intervention. Did you consider Yolanda's goals when doing this?

Performance Patterns

8. What roles have been affected most by Yolanda's fractured humerus?

9. What routines have been affected by her injury?

10. What is the role of OT in addressing Yolanda's roles and routines?

11. Yolanda has a history of alcohol abuse. Is this important to know and, if so, why?

12. What barriers do you see to working with Yolanda?

13. What strengths does Yolanda bring to therapy?

Performance Skills

14. Identify 10 performance skills that are barriers to Yolanda's occupational performance.

15. Identify 10 performance skills that will support her OT intervention.

16. What are Yolanda's self-care deficits, and how would you address these in an outpatient setting?

17. Yolanda is unable to apply her eye makeup, eye shadow, eyeliner, and mascara because she needs both hands to do this. Which specific performance skills is she having difficulty with?

18. How might you address these grooming tasks?

Client Factors

19. Identify key personal and temporal contexts to consider for assessment and intervention.

20. What cultural factors might be important to consider for your intervention planning? Why?

21. According to the physician's initial orders, what types of exercises would you do with Yolanda during the first week? Why would you do them?

22. When would you test the AROM of Yolanda's left UE?

23. Would you give Yolanda activities/exercises for her left hand? Why or why not?

24. Yolanda's physician ordered AROM and AROM activities starting at week 2. Write a home exercise program for Yolanda that follows these physician orders.

25. What type of intervention activities would you start doing in week 2? Please choose four and explain why you chose them. Are these occupation or activity methods of interventions? If your intervention was a preparatory method or task, change it to an activity- or occupation-based one. What type of tools or equipment would you need to implement this intervention?

26. At 3 weeks post-fracture, Yolanda becomes very teary during her intervention sessions, but will not open up to tell you why. How would you handle this?

27. Yolanda tells you that she continues to take Percocet (oxycodone HCL/acetaminophen) three times a day because she is afraid of having pain. Should this concern you? If so, why and what would you do about it?

28. What patient education will Yolanda need in relation to her fracture?

29. Would you use any physical agent modalities during Yolanda's sessions? If so, which ones and why?

Contexts and Environment

30. Identify personal and temporal factors that may influence your assessment and intervention planning.

31. What types of difficulties do you anticipate Yolanda might have at mealtime? What adaptive equipment would you recommend, and how much would it cost?

32. What types of difficulties do you anticipate Yolanda might have with dressing and showering? What adaptive equipment would you recommend, and how much would it cost?

33. Are there any safety concerns regarding Yolanda's ability to function at home?

Theory and Evidence

34. What theory/theories or frame(s) of reference might you use in developing an intervention plan? Describe the rationale for your choices.

35. What, if any, evidence can you find to support your choice of theory/theories and/or frame(s) of reference?

36. What, if any, evidence can you find to support intervention?

Intervention Plan and Goals

37. Are there other assessments you would like to administer? Why? Are they body structure based or occupation based?

38. What would be your long- and short-term goals for Yolanda? Write an intervention plan for Yolanda based on a 3-week timetable.

Situations

39. Yolanda spends a lot of her leisure time socializing and feels the sling she has been given looks ugly; she has decided not to wear it. She says that she can hold her arm still. How would you address this issue?

40. By the third week of intervention, Yolanda has missed her first two appointments. When you call her to see why, she says that she is doing the exercises and that she has more to do to get ready for her trip in 1 week. How would you handle this? Is it important for her to come in for the next two appointments? Why or why not?

41. Yolanda has told you that she has not taken a shower yet because she is afraid of the pain when her arm is out of the sling. How could you work with her on this so that the outcome is that she takes a shower at home?

42. Yolanda usually wears her hair pulled back off her face. She is frustrated that she cannot wear it this way; it makes her feel unkempt. How would you address this issue?

Discharge Planning

43. Yolanda is ready to be discharged. Her arm has just come out of the sling, and she and her husband are leaving on their trip next week. She is still very weak in her left shoulder, and her gross motor coordination is mildly impaired due to the shoulder weakness. What type of program would you give her on discharge, and what would your discharge instructions to her be?

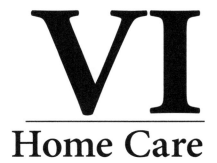

VI
Home Care

18

Alice: Multiple Sclerosis

OCCUPATIONAL PROFILE

Alice is a 51-year-old divorced White woman with a diagnosis of multiple sclerosis (MS). She was diagnosed with MS 18 years ago. In addition, she also has a history of hypertension and recently has had several falls. Her doctor referred her to the Visiting Nurse Association (VNA). Alice had no hospitalization leading to her referral to the home health agency. Her doctor was concerned about the progression of the disease and Alice's ability to manage safely in her home. Alice has been independent in ADLs and IADLs; however, her ex-husband, Jim, who continues to help her with home maintenance tasks, feels that she is not managing meal preparation, laundry, or housekeeping as well as she used to. Alice feels she is doing fine, and there are no changes.

Alice lives in a two-story home in a rural area. The home has a master bedroom and bathroom on the second floor, along with one more bedroom. The first floor has a kitchen, living/family room, half bath, and dining room. Alice retired 2 years ago from her position as a middle school teacher. She found the work too draining and physically demanding. She misses working with the children and being involved in the community. She has two grown daughters, both of whom live out of state. She talks with them occasionally on the phone. Alice used to have a beautiful garden, but has not been able to keep it up over the past few years. She also likes to read magazines and newspapers.

Alice is an independent woman with a strong personality. She comes across as confident and sure of herself. She tends to minimize the impact her disease has had on her life and feels her doctor is "overreacting" in getting the VNA involved in her care. She will be seen by OT and PT for evaluation of ADLs, IADLs, and safety. She has private insurance, but it only covers 20 lifetime OT visits.

ANALYSIS OF OCCUPATIONAL PERFORMANCE

OT evaluation was completed using chart review, interview, observation of functional activity, cognitive assessment using the Behavior Rating Inventory of Executive Function—Adult (BRIEF-A; Roth, Isquith, & Gioia, 2005) and motor assessment. The results of the OT evaluation indicate that Alice has no perceptual, visual, or hearing deficits. She has decreased sensation to touch in her hands.

Lowenstein NA, Halloran P.
Case Studies Through the Health Care Continuum:
A Workbook for the Occupational Therapy Student, Second Edition (pp 81-84).
© 2015 SLACK Incorporated.

She reports a "numb" feeling in both hands, but states that it seems worse at some times than at others. Alice has limited AROM in both shoulders as a result of weakness. Her shoulder AROM is as follows: 100 degrees flexion; 80 degrees abduction; 20 degrees extension; 35 degrees external rotation; 75 degrees internal rotation; 0 degrees horizontal abduction; 55 degrees horizontal adduction; 110 degrees elbow flexion. All other AROM of UEs are within normal limits. She has decreased gross and fine motor coordination, especially as she becomes fatigued. She is able to engage in a task before fatiguing for about 15 minutes. She ambulates with Lofstrand crutches and appears to put a lot of her body weight through her arms to the device. She performs transfers from bed and chair independently, albeit precariously. Her sitting balance is good; her standing balance is fair for static and poor for dynamic with the crutches.

Alice is able to shower and dress herself, but it takes her about 50 minutes to complete her morning routine, and she feels tired by the time she is dressed. She likes to dress nicely every day and wears classic-style clothing—cardigan sweaters, crisp button-down shirts, pleated dress pants, and loafers. Currently, Alice is using a stall shower to bathe. She demonstrates shower transfers as follows: She leaves the crutches outside the shower stall, steps in over the lip of the shower, holding onto the shower faucet to pull herself in, and leans herself in the right corner to help her keep her balance. She gets out by reaching around the shower door for the sink to pull herself out. "I've been doing it like this for a long time. . . no problems!" Alice says.

Alice fatigues quickly, but pushes herself to do as much as possible before "crashing for several hours on the couch." She does all the cooking and laundry and says it sometimes takes her all day just to get the laundry done. The washer and dryer are in the basement, and the stairs leading down are narrow. Alice refuses to demonstrate how she gets downstairs into the basement. "I manage!" she says.

Alice states she makes dinner each night. She uses the oven "carefully." Alice's ex-husband reports that he has noticed that she has a difficult time getting dinner ready and doing most tasks. Alice denies that there is any difference, but he says that he often comes by the house and finds that she has not prepared dinner, but has instead completed parts of different tasks, such as cutting some of the vegetables, or the potatoes are in water on the stove, but the stove is not turned on. She might start cleaning a room, but leave the dust cloths or vacuum in the room without finishing what she started. She will go to the grocery store and just buy food without knowing what is still at home, so she has to throw out a lot of food that has not been used. Results of the BRIEF-A self-report demonstrate difficulty with planning and organization, task monitoring, and initiation and working memory.

Alice is skeptical about receiving OT and does not see how it applies to her. However, she is very clear about PT because she would like to walk more easily "without these bloody crutches!" Her goals are to "keep doing what I'm doing."

QUESTIONS

Occupations

1. Identify which occupations have been most affected by Alice's MS? Why?

2. Given that Alice does not feel she has any issues, how would you prioritize which occupations to begin to address during intervention?

3. Do you feel that OT should address the area of sleep? Why or why not?

Performance Patterns

4. What routines have been affected by Alice's MS diagnosis? How have these routine(s) been affected?

5. What roles have been affected and how would your OT intervention address these roles?

6. How does fatigue affect Alice's daily routines, and how would you address this issue?

Performance Skills

7. Identify 10 key performance skills that are impeding Alice's ability to engage in meaningful occupations.

8. Identify 10 key performance skills that are currently supporting Alice's ability to engage in meaningful occupations.

9. What changes could you suggest for Alice's bathing routine?

10. What changes could you suggest to make Alice's dressing routine easier?

11. What alternative could you suggest to Alice if she feels too fatigued by late afternoon to prepare the evening meal? What could Alice do for meals if her symptoms are interfering with her ability to cook safely?

12. Alice loves to garden and misses being able to get out into her yard to tend to her flowers. She asks you for suggestions to help her resume her hobby.

13. Alice also loves to read while sitting in her reclining chair, but gets tired from holding the newspaper open. She complains that she misses out on the news and asks if you have any suggestions.

14. What safety issues do you see regarding Alice's present routines?

15. What things could Alice do differently to prevent any injury during her routines?

Client Factors

16. Identify important values and beliefs that could influence your OT intervention.

17. Identify 10 key body structures that are impeding Alice's ability to engage in meaningful occupations.

18. Identify 10 key body structures that support her ability to engage in meaningful occupations.

19. What functional activities could you recommend to work on UE strength and ROM?

20. Why might Alice have been reluctant at first to engage in OT intervention?

Contexts and Environment

21. Identify social supports for Alice.

22. Identify key personal and temporal contexts to consider for assessment and intervention.

23. What adaptive equipment might Alice benefit from to increase her independence and safety at home?

24. Using a medical/therapy supply catalogue, determine the total costs of these items.

25. Prioritize the equipment you think Alice needs most if she has only $200 to spend on supplies.

26. What could you do to help adapt Alice's environment cost free?

Theory and Evidence

27. What theory/theories or frame(s) of reference might you use in developing an intervention plan? Describe the rationale for your choice(s).

28. What, if any, evidence can you find to support your choice of theory/theories and/or frame(s) of reference?

29. What, if any, evidence can you find to support intervention?

Intervention Plan and Goals

30. Explain OT to Alice in your own words.

31. Do you feel the COPM would be a good assessment to complete with Alice? Why or why not?

32. What other functional assessment(s) might you consider completing?

33. What would you and Alice set as long-term goals?

34. What would you and Alice set as short-term goals for OT intervention?

35. Write out the intervention plan you would establish for Alice, including frequency of visit.

Situations

36. You arrive at Alice's house for a visit, and she calls for you to come in. As you enter the kitchen (Figure 18-1), you find Alice carrying a chicken pot pie with one hand and trying to hold onto the counter for balance with the other. The food is obviously hot as the kitchen has a fresh-baked aroma. How do you address this safety concern with Alice? List several ways and her possible reactions to your comments.

37. Assume that, after you mention this to Alice, she becomes defensive and tells you she is not a child. How would you deal with her feelings?

38. You arrive at Alice's home, and she is visibly shaken. She tells you that she fell about 45 minutes ago and just got herself up onto the kitchen chair. She tells you she feels fine and she is just "mad at herself" for getting stuck between the counter and the kitchen table. She says, "It could happen to anyone!" What would you do? Alice tells you not to mention the fall to the physical therapist or anyone else. What would you say?

39. You arrive at Alice's house for a scheduled visit. There is no answer at the door, and it is locked as always. She has never missed a visit before. You are worried she may have fallen and is unable to get to the door. What would you do?

40. You arrive at Alice's home and there is no answer when you knock, but the front door is unlocked. You go in and find Alice on the bathroom floor. She says she has pain in her shoulder and tells you to help her up. What would you do?

41. What could be done to improve Alice's safety during ambulation? What could be instituted so she could be safer while alone?

42. Alice's ex-husband comes by one day during your session. He asks you what he can do to help Alice. She shouts out, "Nothing! I'm fine! This is my problem." What would you tell him?

Discharge Planning

43. You have met all your goals with Alice and plan to discontinue OT. However, because of the nature of her disease, you know that it is likely that she will need further intervention. How would you explain to her the need to discontinue OT?

44. How can you be assured that Alice will get the OT interventions needed once that situation arises?

Figure 18-1. Alice's kitchen.

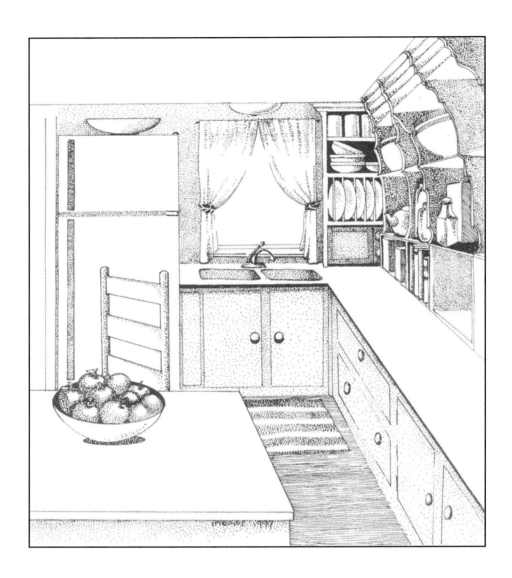

REFERENCE

Roth, R. M., Isquith, P. K., & Gioia, G. A. (2005). *Behavior Rating Inventory of Executive Function—Adult Version*. Lutz, FL: Psychological Assessment Resources.

19

Barb: Left Cerebrovascular Accident, Right Hemiparesis, and Expressive Aphasia

OCCUPATIONAL PROFILE

Barb is a 72-year-old White woman with a diagnosis of left CVA with subsequent right hemiparesis and expressive aphasia. She has secondary diagnoses of hypertension, a hysterectomy 12 years ago, and a history of transient ischemic attacks (TIAs). Barb was hospitalized 2 months ago when her son noticed that she had a right-sided facial droop and took her to the emergency department. She spent 2 weeks in the community hospital and was then transferred for a 4-week stay at an area rehabilitation hospital. She was discharged home from there.

Barb lives alone in a small studio apartment in a senior apartment complex. Her apartment is on the third floor of an elevator building. The common rooms, mail, and laundry are all on the first floor. She has been widowed for 21 years and is used to taking care of herself and her own affairs. She retired 7 years ago from a position she had held for 32 years as a receptionist at a downtown law firm.

Barb has two sons, both of whom are married and living in nearby communities. She sees each of them about twice a month because her sons both work long hours and are busy with their jobs and families. She has only one sibling—a

sister, Beatrice—who lives in Florida. Barb visits her for the month of February each year.

Barb was very active before the onset of her CVA. She went out with friends daily and participated in the senior outings in her building. She always went on the monthly bus trips they offered, with her favorite being to the casino. She volunteered 2 hours a week at a soup kitchen where she served meals to the homeless, and she liked to read to the children in the day care that is housed in her building. She walked indoors at the YMCA and covered approximately 2 miles three times a week. Occasionally, Barb would babysit for her grandchildren, aged 3 and 7, but reportedly expressed the sentiment, "I'm too old for that . . . I've done my child raising already!" She enjoyed reading magazines, especially home and women's magazines. Barb never learned to drive and instead took public transportation everywhere she needed to go. She was independent in all of her daily tasks before the onset of the CVA.

Barb reluctantly came home from the rehabilitation hospital. Reportedly, she is unsure of her ability to manage at home and is afraid of failing and being put into a nursing home. However, her biggest concern is how to face her friends again. She is very embarrassed about her expressive aphasia and declined all of their visits and phone calls while

Lowenstein NA, Halloran P.
Case Studies Through the Health Care Continuum:
A Workbook for the Occupational Therapy Student, Second Edition (pp 85-88).
© 2015 SLACK Incorporated.

she was in the hospital and rehabilitation facility. The discharge plan is for Barb to remain in her own apartment and manage safely with community health support services. She was referred to the VNA for nursing, PT, OT, speech therapy, and home health aide services. She has Medicare Parts A and B.

ANALYSIS OF OCCUPATIONAL PERFORMANCE

Barb was evaluated by OT through the discharge notes from the rehabilitation hospital, limited interview because of the expressive aphasia, and observation of functional tasks. During this visit, Barb was somewhat guarded. She becomes frustrated quickly regarding her speech and stops trying to answer questions when she cannot get her point across after the second or third try. It is difficult to formally assess Barb's cognitive function because of her expressive aphasia. Her communication skills are limited by word-finding problems and difficulty articulating even one-word answers. Her vision, hearing, and sensation appear intact on observation. She approaches tasks in a slow, cautious, and disorganized manner. She has good judgment about her skills, but appears to have short retention and attention spans. She has difficulty with new learning and seems to prefer doing things "the old way."

Barb has approximately half of the normal ROM in her right shoulder. Her strength is obviously impaired, and her gross and fine motor coordination is poor. She is unable to fully grasp or maintain a grasp on any items, rendering her right arm nonfunctional. Barb is able to oppose her thumb to the lateral side of the second and third digits only. She is inconsistently able to extend all digits. Barb's tone on the right side is 1 on the Ashworth Scale. She is right-hand dominant. She has pain in the right shoulder at the end ranges of all shoulder motions. She scores it a 4 on a visual scale of 1 to 10. She has slight edema in the right hand. She has no AROM deficits or strength deficits in her left UE.

Barb is able to ambulate independently with a small-based quad cane while wearing a right ankle-foot orthosis. She is able to independently transfer from standing to/from her couch. She also transfers independently to/from the over-toilet commode. Her static balance is good; dynamic balance is fair. She has a shower seat and grab bars in her shower. She refuses to demonstrate the shower transfers and looks frightened at the suggestion.

Barb's couch is a pull-out bed. This is where she had been sleeping before the CVA. It appears that now Barb is sleeping on the couch without pulling out the bed.

Barb is able to dress and sponge-bathe herself while sitting at the sink without any adaptive equipment. She uses one-handed techniques for dressing herself. Barb has been wearing sweat suits that one of her son's bought for her when she was in the rehabilitation hospital, but she would prefer to dress in her skirts, shirts, and tops like she used to wear. She becomes tired easily during her morning routine, and it takes her much longer to get ready in the morning than before her stroke. She uses the microwave independently to heat precooked meals her sons bring for her. For convenience, her microwave is on the table where she eats. However, she is unable to open some of the containers her meals are in and has difficulty carrying food from the refrigerator to the microwave. She cannot open cans, bottles, or packages. Barb needs assistance for all home management tasks. She now has to rely on her sons to do all her shopping, laundry, and to pay her bills. Barb is unable to articulate her goals because of her expressive aphasia.

QUESTIONS

Occupations

1. Identify the ADL, IADL, rest/sleep, work, leisure, and social participation occupations most affected by Barb's CVA.

2. Identify the occupations in which Barb can still participate.

3. How would you prioritize these occupations in your intervention planning? Explain your reasoning.

4. What leisure occupation do you feel Barb could resume first? Explain your reasoning.

5. Barb declines to engage in social activities again. Explain the impact you feel this has on her and what could be done to address it.

Performance Patterns

6. How have Barb's routines been affected by her CVA?

7. Which routines have been affected the most? Why?

8. Which routines do you feel should be addressed first by OT? Why? Did you consider Barb's goals?

9. Which roles have been most affected by Barb's CVA? Explain your answer?

10. Do you feel that OT will enable Barb to regain these roles? Which ones? Explain your thinking.

Performance Skills

11. Identify five key motor skills that are having a negative impact on Barb's engagement in occupations.

12. Identify five key process skills that are having a negative impact on Barb's engagement in occupations.

13. Identify five key social interaction skills that are having a negative impact on Barb's engagement in occupations.

14. Identify five key motor performance skills that are supporting Barb's engagement in her current occupations.

15. Identify five key process performance skills that are supporting Barb's engagement in her current occupations.

16. Identify five key social interaction skills that are supporting Barb's engagement in her current occupations.

17. Write a plan to help Barb address her deficits in meal preparation.

18. Given Barb's expressive aphasia, how would you get her perspective on her progress and goals?

Client Factors

19. What body functions are impeding Barb's ability to pull out the bed?

20. What body functions are having an impact on her right UE movement?

21. Identify 10 key body functions that are affecting Barb's performance skills.

22. Identify five key body functions that may be affecting her cognitive skills.

23. What suggestions could you give Barb to manage the edema and pain in her right arm? Why is it important to deal with both of these issues? What could occur if the edema and pain issues are not addressed?

24. Explain which OT intervention method you would use for the hypotonicity in her right arm.

25. Write a home exercise program for Barb.

26. After 2 weeks, Barb shows improvement in the AROM of her right hand. She is able to maintain a grasp on large, lightweight items. What changes, if any, would you make in her intervention plan and/or goals? Why?

27. After 2 weeks, Barb is able to use her hand as a gross assist. What tasks may she now be able to do that she could not before?

28. Given her cognitive status, how would you need to adapt your intervention sessions for Barb?

29. What could you do to be sure Barb is retaining new information?

Contexts and Environment

30. Identify key personal and temporal contexts to consider for assessment and intervention.

31. Identify social supports that may be useful for Barb.

32. How would you address her ability to open her bed for sleeping?

33. Barb occasionally leaves the apartment during the daytime hours to get her mail. However, she will usually do this around 9 p.m. List some reasons why she may do this.

34. What community resources may be helpful for Barb to manage her meals? Find the supports available in her community.

35. What adaptations may help Barb to be more independent? Be specific. Explain why these adaptations would be important.

36. What additional adaptive devices may be useful for her to maximize independence?

37. What problems may arise as you try to train Barb in adaptive equipment use? What type of impact has the CVA had on Barb's family? How has this changed their roles?

38. What are some of the ways you might provide education to Barb?

39. How could you utilize other team members to educate Barb and ensure carryover of intervention?

Theory and Evidence

40. What theory/theories or frame(s) of reference might you use in developing an intervention plan? Describe the rationale for your choice(s).

41. What, if any, evidence can you find to support your choice of theory/theories and/or frame of reference?

42. What, if any, evidence can you find to support intervention?

Intervention Plan and Goals

43. What long-term goals would you and Barb set for her OT intervention?

44. What short-term goals would you and Barb set for OT?

45. What, if any, other assessments would you consider administering, and why?

46. Devise an OT intervention plan for Barb for the first 2 weeks of OT. Be sure to include frequency of intervention.

Situations

47. After a few weeks, you are asked by the case managing nurse to do the home health aide (HHA) supervision visit. The HHA had been scheduled for three times per week. The HHA tells you that Barb refuses showers. She only lets the HHA wash her hair in the sink. List three reasons that Barb might be refusing showers. What would you suggest as a solution for each of these reasons?

48. Do you think Barb should continue to have an HHA three times a week? Please explain your answer.

49. How could you focus your intervention sessions so that Barb no longer needs the HHA?

50. One day, after 20 minutes of intervention, Barb becomes discouraged about her inability to communicate. She waves you off, gets up from the table, and walks away from you. How would you handle this?

51. How would you handle it if this behavior occurred for several sessions?

52. Barb's sister, Beatrice, wants her to come to visit for the month of February as she usually does. What are some issues Barb should address before taking her trip?

53. Barb is upset after she returns from a doctor's appointment. The doctor told her that her hand would never be normal. She is teary and upset. She tells you not to come anymore because it is not worth it. What would you do in this situation?

Discharge Planning

54. At what point would you decide to discharge Barb from OT services? How would you know it is time for discharge?

55. Given that Barb does not want OT to end, how would you go about discharging her from service? Write a discharge note to Barb's doctor.

Dmitri: Right Distal Radial and Ulnar Fracture

OCCUPATIONAL PROFILE

Dmitri is a 92-year-old Russian-speaking man who lives in an assisted living facility. He fell in his bathroom and fractured his right distal radius and ulna. He was sent to the emergency department. X-rays revealed a clean fracture with no need for surgery to stabilize the fractures. His arm was placed in a full arm cast with elbow in flexion in the emergency department, and he was sent back to the assistive living facility. He has a history of non–insulin-dependent diabetes, congestive heart failure, cataracts, and alcohol abuse. He did have his left cataract removed several years ago, but his right cataract cannot be removed because of macular degeneration in that eye.

Dmitri lives in a first-floor apartment and has to go up the elevator to the dining room on the fourth floor. He is widowed and has a son who is in a nursing home with Parkinson's disease; he had another son who passed away at age 70 from a heart attack. He has no other living family. He does not drive, but likes to walk daily, regardless of the weather. He goes out into the neighborhood to get a newspaper and a cup of coffee. Dmitri has a pet bird that he lets out of the cage daily. The bird is trained to go back into its cage when Dmitri tells it to. He is fond of his bird. They have "conversations," and Dmitri calls the bird "his family." The assisted living staff does his meals and laundry and, because of his limited English, he is not able to participate in many of the assisted living activities. He enjoys reading his Russian-language newspapers and books. In Russia, Dmitri had been a farmer. The hard work took a toll on his body, and he has many aches and pains in his knees, back, and neck.

Dmitri came to this country 20 years ago to be near his sons. He did not learn English. He knows some common phrases, such as "how are you?" and "I am fine," but is not conversational. He lived with his son before the son's nursing home placement. Dmitri is not able to care for his son and feels guilty that he cannot care for him or see him often. The nursing home is too far to walk, and there is no public transportation to get there. Dmitri has to rely on a volunteer from senior services to take him there every other week, but doctor appointments take priority, so he never knows when they will call him to offer the ride.

Dmitri is a fiercely independent man who lived through a great deal in his Russian homeland. He does not like to ask for help, and he has a difficult time accepting help from others. He is being seen in home care by nursing and OT.

Lowenstein NA, Halloran P.
Case Studies Through the Health Care Continuum:
A Workbook for the Occupational Therapy Student, Second Edition (pp 89-91).
© 2015 SLACK Incorporated.

It is difficult to ascertain what his goal is because of the language barrier.

ANALYSIS OF OCCUPATIONAL PERFORMANCE

Dmitri was evaluated by chart review, limited interview because of the language barrier, and motor assessment. Dmitri's cognition appears intact but, again, it is difficult to assess because of the language barrier. He has no significant perceptual deficits. He wears glasses, and his vision is poor in his right eye because of his cataract. Sensation in his hands is decreased for sharp–dull; and he complains of numbness and tingling in his right hand, especially his fingers. His right UE cast has just been removed. He has strength in his left UE of 4/5 throughout. His right UE has 4/5 in shoulder movements, but 3+/5 in the elbow and hand and 3–/5 in his wrist. His has edema of the wrist and fingers, and he complains of pain with most wrist movements. He has AROM in his elbow of minus 25-degree extension; in his wrist of 20-degree flexion and 15-degree extension. His fingers are minus one-third of full range of movement. His coordination is impaired for fine motor and dexterity tasks with his right UE, but intact for the left UE. His gross motor coordination is mildly impaired on the right UE because of his decreased elbow AROM; his left is within functional limits. Dmitri is right-handed.

Dmitri is independent in all transfers. He can shower with moderate assistance and dresses his upper and lower body with minimal assistance. Fasteners are difficult for him to do. He cannot tie his shoes, and he requires minimum assistance to button his shirt and zip his slacks. Dmitri ambulates with a rollator walker that he has difficulty using because of his injury. He has difficulty holding the newspaper and gets frustrated, but will not ask for more help from anyone. He looks forward to OT so that he can "get better."

QUESTIONS

Occupation

1. What are the ADL occupations most affected by Dmitri's fracture?

2. Identify five other occupations (not ADL) that are affected by his injury.

3. How would you address Dmitri's engagement in leisure activities?

4. Do you feel it is important for Dmitri to become more involved in the activities in the assisted living residence? Why?

Performance Patterns

5. What routines have been most affected by Dmitri's injury? In what ways?

6. What roles have been affected by his injury?

7. Why is it important to understand Dmitri's roles, routines, and habits for OT?

Performance Skills

8. Identify 10 key performance skills that are impeding Dmitri's performance in his desired occupations. Explain your choices.

9. Identify 10 key performance skills that support his current performance in his desired occupations. Explain your choices.

10. How would you address Dmitri's bathing deficits?

11. How would you address his dressing deficits?

Client Factors

12. Identify 10 key body structures that would support your OT intervention.

13. Identify 10 key body structures that are barriers to Dmitri's current occupational engagement.

14. What safety issues would you want to be aware of when working with Dmitri? How would you explain these to Dmitri so that he understands them?

15. Write a home exercise program for Dmitri to follow. How would you do this so that he understands the exercises?

16. What functional activities could you do to increase Dmitri's AROM and strength in his right wrist and elbow?

17. Given his decreased hand dexterity and fine motor coordination, write a plan for an intervention session for each of the intervention methods (preparatory methods/tasks, activity and occupation).

18. Change the activities listed in Question 17 to account for improvement in his dexterity and fine motor skills.

19. How would you address Dmitri's decreased sensation? What are important safety concerns for this deficit?

20. Given that your home health agency has a small budget for supplies and does not provide Thera-Band (The Hygenic Corp), Thera-Putty (GF Health Products, Inc), or any other exercise equipment, what common household objects could you use for improving strength?

21. How would you address the edema in Dmitri's hand and wrist?

22. Dmitri has a poor memory and forgets to take his medication and perform his daily exercises and cannot remember where he has put commonly used items, like his eyeglasses, keys, and wallet. How could OT address these issues?

23. Dmitri is fiercely independent and resists most of your ideas about help and changes to his routine and environment. How could you address these issues?

Contexts and Environment

24. What aspects of Dmitri's cultural background would be important for you to understand? How would you go about understanding his cultural background?

25. Given Dmitri's limited knowledge of English, how would you communicate with him?

26. Given Dmitri's memory deficits and cultural issues, how would you address patient education?

27. What, if any, adaptive equipment do you feel Dmitri might benefit from for his bathing and dressing? What is the cost of this equipment?

28. Dmitri likes to keep his lights low, so he uses low wattage bulbs in his apartment and does not like to turn on the lights. You suspect this may have contributed to his fall. How would you approach Dmitri to encourage him to address these issues?

Theory and Evidence

29. What theory/theories or frame(s) of reference might you use in developing an intervention plan? Describe the rationale for your choice(s).

30. What, if any, evidence can you find to support your choice of theory/theories and/or frame(s) of reference?

31. What, if any, evidence can you find to support intervention?

Intervention Plan and Goals

32. Given that Dmitri is unable to tell you his goals, how would you develop a problem list and prioritize it?

33. What are Dmitri's deficits in the occupational performance area of instrumental ADL? Can you make some assumptions about the difficulties he might have in areas that are not specifically mentioned in the evaluation?

34. Are there other assessments that you would like to administer and, if so, why?

35. Write a list of long- and short-term goals addressing bathing and dressing.

36. Write a list of functional long- and short-term goals to address Dmitri's UE status.

Situations

37. You have been starting off your intervention sessions with a few minutes of exercises. Today, when you do this, Dmitri complains of pain in his wrist. You feel it and notice it is warm to touch and slightly swollen. What would you do and why? What types of activities would you do that would not exacerbate his wrist pain?

38. Dmitri's wrist has healed in a poorly aligned position. He complains of wrist pain when he wakes in the morning and of numbness and tingling in his hands. What do you think might be the cause of this, and what would you do?

Discharge Planning

39. Dmitri has achieved all but a few goals. He still does not have full AROM in his wrist and fingers, but they are now functional. Would you recommend outpatient therapy for him?

40. How would you arrange to get Dmitri to outpatient therapy?

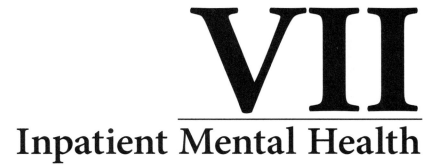

VII
Inpatient Mental Health

Elizabeth: Major Depressive Disorder With Suicide Attempt

OCCUPATIONAL PROFILE

Elizabeth is a 25-year-old woman with a diagnosis of major depression with a suicide attempt by overdose of acetaminophen and codeine. She was sent to the hospital emergency department from her college's health services, where her roommate had taken her when she found her unconscious in their room. Elizabeth had stopped eating and had been having difficulty concentrating on her studies. She is in her last year of law school. She had been doing well until she and her girlfriend of 4 years, Susan, broke up. They met during their sophomore year at college and had been together ever since. Elizabeth assumed they would move in together after their graduations and start a life together. They had applied to all the same law schools and decided which one to go to together. Law school was difficult for Elizabeth, and she had to spend more time in the law library than with Susan. Because of this, they did not see each other as much as either would have liked. Elizabeth was surprised when Susan told her that she had met someone else and that she felt it would be better if they broke up. Elizabeth felt that if she were smarter and did not have to study so much, none of this would have happened.

Elizabeth grew up in a large city as the youngest of three children. Her mother died from breast cancer when she was 13, and her father remarried 18 months later. Elizabeth did not get along with her stepmother and was thrilled to go as far away from her family as she could for college. Her father supports her during graduate school, and she gets summer jobs to pay for books, clothes, and entertainment. Elizabeth has two older brothers, with whom she is fairly close, but they live in different states; she talks to them by phone or Skype (Microsoft) when she can, and they text pretty regularly.

Before her suicide attempt, Elizabeth had been living in an apartment with Susan and another roommate for 2 years. They shared all the cooking and chores of the apartment. She works hard at school and maintains a B average. She is looking forward to finishing and working in family law. Elizabeth is a hardworking, driven person. She feels that she has to prove to her older brothers and father that she is a capable person in her own right and that they do not have to protect her. She was close to her mother, and her death was difficult for her.

Elizabeth is in the locked unit on suicide precautions. The milieu team is seeing her and is composed of a social worker, psychiatric nurse, and occupational therapist, as

Lowenstein NA, Halloran P.
Case Studies Through the Health Care Continuum:
A Workbook for the Occupational Therapy Student, Second Edition (pp 95-97).
© 2015 SLACK Incorporated.

well as her psychiatrist. Her expected length of stay is 1 to 2 weeks, with discharge back to her apartment.

ANALYSIS OF OCCUPATIONAL PERFORMANCE

Elizabeth was evaluated by OT the morning after she was admitted from the emergency department. OT evaluation was completed through interview and observation of her on the unit. She appeared disheveled; her hair was uncombed, and her clothes were unkempt. Her affect was flat and she made little eye contact. She spoke softly and looked down when she talked. Elizabeth had difficulty thinking of interests because everything that she thought about were activities that she and Susan had done together, and she cries at these thoughts. Elizabeth mentions that they camped together and liked the outdoors, movies, and reading. She cannot think of activities that she did by herself before she met Susan. She speaks about wanting to join her mother, "now that she has lost everything worthwhile in her life." She is on suicide precautions with checks every 15 minutes. Her expected length of stay is 2 weeks, with discharge expected back to her own apartment. Although pessimistic about her ability to do so, Elizabeth is motivated by a desire to get out of the hospital in time to return to school to finish her last year with her class. Finals for the first semester are in 1 month, and her goal is to be able to take these with her classmates.

QUESTIONS

Occupations

1. Identity five key occupations that OT should address during Elizabeth's hospital stay. Explain your reason for choosing these occupations.

2. Elizabeth had difficulty identifying leisure interests during the OT evaluation. How could you explore this with her, and what might you suggest, given what you know about her? Are there any additional assessments you might administer to assist Elizabeth in identifying leisure interests?

3. Elizabeth is determined to finish law school with her class, despite the fact that she is missing 2 weeks of classes and had been falling behind for 3 weeks before her hospitalization. How can you help her address this issue?

4. Elizabeth's roommate comes to visit and brings her some clothes and makeup. Elizabeth refuses to put on her makeup, saying "there is no one worth looking pretty for." She wears the same clothes that she came in with and refuses to change them. How could you and the team address this issue?

5. During a conversation with Elizabeth, you discover that she enjoys cooking gourmet meals. What could you do with this information? What if there is a kitchen on the unit? What if there is no kitchen on the unit?

Performance Patterns

6. Describe which roles have been disrupted and the impact of this disruption on Elizabeth's engagement in occupations.

7. Do you feel there is one role loss that has affected Elizabeth's engagement in occupations more than others? How could you use her student role to return to some of her routines?

8. What routines have been affected by Elizabeth's depression? What do you hypothesize is the reason for the disruption of her routines?

Performance Skills

9. Identify 10 key performance skills that are having a negative impact on Elizabeth's engagement in meaningful occupations.

10. Identify 10 key performance skills that you would consider strengths of Elizabeth's that you might incorporate into your intervention.

11. Take three to five of your identified performance skills from Questions 9 and 10 and create a group intervention that can address these.

Client Factors

12. Identify 10 key body functions that are affecting Susan's engagement in occupations.

13. Identify 10 key body functions that could be considered strengths for OT intervention.

14. Identify three values that you feel are important to Elizabeth. Explain your thinking. How might you use this information in developing your OT intervention?

Contexts and Environment

15. Identify key personal and temporal contexts to consider for assessment and intervention.

16. What cultural considerations would you consider in developing your intervention? Why?

17. What are some social supports that you can identify for Elizabeth upon discharge? How would you start to put these in place before her discharge?

18. Do you feel it would be a good idea for Elizabeth to return to the same apartment that she shared with Susan? Why or why not?

19. How would you educate Elizabeth about her diagnosis and the stress she will be under when she leaves the hospital?

20. Given that Elizabeth is on suicide precautions, what safety issues would you have to be aware of during OT intervention?

Theory and Evidence

21. What theory/theories or frame(s) of reference might you use in developing an intervention plan? Describe the rationale for your choice(s).

22. What, if any, evidence can you find to support your choice of theory/theories and/or frame(s) of reference?

23. What, if any, evidence can you find to support intervention?

Intervention Plan and Goals

24. Identify assessments that you might administer to complete your evaluation. Why did you choose these?

25. Write out a problem list based on Elizabeth's evaluation and history.

26. Given Elizabeth's goals, what long- and short-term goals you would set up with her?

27. What obstacles do you anticipate Elizabeth might face in reaching these goals in the expected time frame?

28. What strengths can you identify that might assist Elizabeth in reaching her goals?

29. What groups do you feel Elizabeth would benefit from? Explain your reasoning.

Situations

30. It is the second week of Elizabeth's hospitalization, and she has been showing signs of improving. You have just finished an arts and crafts group that required the patients to use scissors, and you find that there is a pair of scissors missing. Elizabeth left the room quickly after the group ended, and you suspect she might have taken them. What would you do?

31. Continuing from Question 30, you have talked to Elizabeth about the scissors, and she has flatly denied taking them. She gets angry with you and says she is going to report you for harassing her. You feel confident that Elizabeth has the scissors. What would you do?

32. Elizabeth talks daily with her father, who wants her to come home for the rest of the semester. Elizabeth tells him she will not do this, but he keeps insisting. She tells you this and asks what she should do. She has not talked about this with any other team members. What would you do?

33. Elizabeth has been coming to life skills group every day for 1 week. Your goal is to have her start making choices about the tasks she wishes to complete and to do some problem solving. She has been having a difficult time making choices and keeps asking you to tell her what to do. How could you assist her in this area?

Discharge Planning

34. After 2 weeks of inpatient hospitalization and medication, Elizabeth is ready to be discharged back to her apartment and to return to school. She is taking care of her grooming, dressing, and hygiene again and expresses that she is happy to be leaving the hospital. She is worried about catching up on the work she missed and is concerned about what she will do the first time she sees Susan in class (she cannot avoid this because they are taking the same classes). Write a discharge note to send to the university's health service.

35. What supports would you recommend for Elizabeth upon discharge?

22

Fred: Schizophrenia, Paranoid With Acute Psychosis

Occupational Profile

Fred is a 19-year-old White man with a diagnosis of paranoid schizophrenia with acute psychosis. Fred has no other diagnoses in his medical history and has been hospitalized only once before because of his schizophrenia. Fred lives with his mother, Karen, in an apartment in the suburbs.

Fred was admitted to the psychiatric unit from the emergency department of the hospital. His two older brothers, Jerry and Joey, brought him into the hospital at the request of their mother. Fred had been becoming gradually more psychotic over the past 2 weeks. His symptoms culminated with him locking himself in the bedroom over several days and refusing to let anyone in. Fred believes his employer is trying to kill him. He had gathered multiple objects in his room to protect himself, including a knife, a baseball bat, and a hammer and refused to let his mother answer the telephone; he insisted they keep all the shades drawn and the lights dimmed.

Fred has been experiencing auditory hallucinations. He claims he can hear his deceased father telling him to "Watch out!" and "Look behind you!" Fred says his father once told him to kill his employer, if needed, to protect

himself. Fred's brother Jerry convinced him to come out of his room to the car only by telling him that their father told Jerry to bring Fred to a safer place. He was seen in the emergency department and admitted to the mental health unit of the hospital.

Fred's symptoms began after he was suspended from work. Fred has been working at a distribution house where he loads boxed items into trucks. He had been an employee for only 3 months. Fred reported that one of his coworkers told him to move boxes from the warehouse to the loading dock using the forklift. His coworker gave him a quick demonstration and then left the area. Fred attempted to move the boxes with the lift and instead ran them over, causing several thousand dollars worth of damage. Fred did not have to pay the company back but was suspended without pay for 2 days. This was 2.5 weeks ago. Fred has not returned to work since.

Fred had his first psychotic episode when he was 17 and started to take medication that managed his symptoms well. He finished high school but did not want to go to college. In high school, he did not have many friends, and his interests were limited to the photography club. Since high school, he has held several jobs, but has not been able to keep one for longer than 6 months. Fred was admitted to the inpatient unit of the hospital. Fred was unable to state

Lowenstein NA, Halloran P.
Case Studies Through the Health Care Continuum:
A Workbook for the Occupational Therapy Student, Second Edition (pp 99-101).
© 2015 SLACK Incorporated.

any goals upon his admission; however, his mother would like him to be able to live on his own and hold a job. Fred's psychiatrist is a physician on the unit and plans to follow his care. Fred will be involved in groups on the unit, and the team consists of his psychiatrist, nursing, social work, OT, and art therapy. He is insured through his mother's insurance company, which covers a maximum of 30 inpatient days for mental health issues.

ANALYSIS OF OCCUPATIONAL PERFORMANCE

Fred is seen by the occupational therapist after he has been on the unit for 1 day. An observation of Fred reveals him to be somewhat unkempt. His clothes are wrinkled and dirty; his hands are also dirty, and he is unshaven. His hair is short, but tousled and looks as though it needs to be washed. Fred appears to be neglecting his basic self-care.

Upon approach, Fred is guarded and minimally verbal. He makes no eye contact and looks down at the floor or at the wall during his meeting with the occupational therapist. He wrings his hands together constantly and rocks his body back and forth slightly in the chair. "I don't want to talk to you!" he barks loudly after introductions. He gets up, looks around, then returns and sits down in the same seat again. "Go away!" he says in a low, stern voice. "GO AWAY!" Fred then leaves the group area for his room. Thus, the evaluation could not be completed.

QUESTIONS

Occupations

1. Identify the key occupations that have been affected by Fred's illness.

2. Discuss how Fred's schizophrenia may have affected the development of other occupations as a teen and why.

3. How would you prioritize the occupations to address during Fred's inpatient stay? Why did you put them in the order you did?

4. As an occupational therapist, how might you address the occupation of work? Describe your reasoning.

Performance Patterns

5. Do you feel that Fred had well-established routines and roles before his hospitalization? If so, what were they? If not, what were the barriers preventing the development of routines and roles?

6. How can OT intervention address Fred's routines and roles?

Performance Skills

7. Describe the performance skills that have a positive impact on Fred's engagement in occupation.

8. Describe the performance skills that could be barriers to his engagement in occupation.

9. How might OT assist Fred with improving his ability to perform his ADLs? Explain.

10. What are some of the social skills that Fred is currently unable to demonstrate?

Client Factors

11. What are important values and beliefs to consider during your assessment and intervention? How did you identify these?

12. Identify 10 key body functions that are negatively affecting Fred's engagement in occupations.

13. Identify 10 key body functions that are positively affecting his engagement in occupations.

14. Describe the cognitive deficits Fred's psychosis has caused.

15. Given what you know about Fred, what level do you think he would be at, according to the Allen Cognitive Disability Levels? Why?

16. According to the Model of Human Occupation, what are Fred's strengths and deficits?

Contexts and Environment

17. Identify key personal and temporal contexts to consider for assessment and intervention.

18. What are current social supports to consider during your assessment and intervention?

19. What are some precautions the staff could take when approaching Fred?

20. What impact do you think Fred's illness has had on his mother? On his brothers?

21. What are some safety concerns for Fred?

22. What type of adaptations would need to be made to Fred's environment to ensure his safety?

23. What type of adaptive equipment would Fred need to enable him to be more independent in daily tasks?

Theory and Evidence

24. What theory/theories or frame(s) of reference might you use in developing an intervention plan? Describe the rationale for your choice(s).

25. What, if any, evidence can you find to support your choice of theory/theories and/or frame(s) of reference?

26. What, if any, evidence can you find to support intervention?

Intervention Plan and Goals

27. How would you help Fred set goals if he is unable/unwilling to communicate with you at this time?

28. How would you attempt to complete the OT evaluation with Fred?

29. What would you do to get the information needed for the evaluation, or do you have enough information already?

30. Are there other assessments that you feel would be beneficial to administer? If so, why did you choose these? Explain your reasoning.

31. How would you assess Fred's leisure interests?

32. What type of unit activity groups would be appropriate for Fred? Why?

33. What type of unit activities groups would not be appropriate for Fred? Why?

Situations

34. Fred attends community meetings every day at the request of his doctor. What OT groups would you ask Fred to attend? Why?

35. You are in a cooking group and are about to make oatmeal cookies with three other patients. Fred asks to join your group. This is his first time initiating involvement with others. What would you do and why?

36. You are in a community meeting and notice Fred shaking his head intermittently as if he is responding "no" to someone. What would you do?

37. Fred frequently signs out the unit radio and listens to music quietly by himself at the end of the hall. How could you use this information to enhance Fred's intervention plan?

38. Fred continues to be withdrawn and isolated. How would you approach him to increase his socialization? Explain.

39. Fred's doctor wants him to attend a work task group. What questions would you need answered before you begin?

40. How would you set up Fred's workstation to simulate his work? What safety issues would you want to address before beginning the group?

Discharge Planning

41. Fred is to be discharged from the inpatient unit to the day treatment hospital. Would you recommend OT for Fred at the day hospital? Why?

42. What goals do you feel Fred should meet before he is discharged from the hospital?

43. Write a discharge note for Fred.

23

George: Bipolar Disorder

OCCUPATIONAL PROFILE

George is a 37-year-old Black man with a diagnosis of bipolar disorder. George has a secondary diagnosis of alcohol and cocaine abuse and a past medical history of hospitalizations related to his substance abuse and his bipolar disorder. George is admitted to the inpatient treatment facility from the emergency department.

George has reportedly become increasingly manic over the past 3 weeks. His symptoms include extreme talkativeness, flights of ideas, grandiosity, shopping sprees, and lack of sleep. George denies using any illegal substances. This is confirmed by his blood tests. George's wife, Nina, reports he's been taking his medication, lithium, sporadically for more than 1 month.

George has two sons, aged 10 and 8. He is currently separated from his wife, to whom he has been married for 12 years. He and Nina have separated in the past, usually around the time that the mania or the substance abuse has begun. At his request, Nina is contacted when George is admitted to the hospital. She refuses to come to the hospital, but does answer the psychiatrist's questions over the phone. "He stops taking his medication and gets crazy on me! I'm not letting the boys see it anymore.

I'll do what I can to help, but I'm not going down there again!" she says.

George is an educated man with a master's degree in marketing and public relations. He has been trying to get his own business off the ground. Until 2 months ago, George had been working for an investment firm in the marketing department, but felt "confined by the rules of a large corporation." He had been at that job for less than 1 year. George is very good at what he does, but his personality and his unreliability often result in conflicts with management. The pattern usually continues with George either quitting or getting fired. In the last instance, he quit his job with the plan of running his own business full time rather than on a consulting basis. However, his own business is not doing well, simply because he has not been able to stay focused on it long enough to make it run smoothly. Before the exacerbation of his illness, George had been working full time and managing his home and self independently. When he is not experiencing symptoms, he is described as social and fun to be around. He loves his kids and likes to attend their athletic games and the other activities they do. Before he had children, he was a runner and liked to run in local races to raise money for charities. George and his wife met in college. His wife makes it clear that he is not welcome back in their home as long as he is experiencing

Lowenstein NA, Halloran P.
Case Studies Through the Health Care Continuum:
A Workbook for the Occupational Therapy Student, Second Edition (pp 103-106).
© 2015 SLACK Incorporated.

manic symptoms. She expresses that she might not let him back into their home at all.

George's goals are to return to his home with his wife and children and to work on building a successful business. George is to be involved with psychiatry, nursing, recreation, OT, and social work. His expected length of stay is 7 to 10 days.

ANALYSIS OF OCCUPATIONAL PERFORMANCE

Upon approach, George is eager to talk with the occupational therapist. "I've been waiting for you to get to me! When can I start groups?" he shouts down the hall as the OT walks toward him. The therapist leads George into a quiet room. The room has a small table and two chairs. There are large glass windows on either side of the door so the staff can see in and patients can see out. During the evaluation, George has a difficult time remaining in his seat. He gets up and then sits down again frequently. When he is sitting, he is unable to remain still. He picks pieces of lint off the chair, kicks the table leg, and twists the phone cord until the receiver falls off the hook.

George is unable to stay focused on the conversation. His speech is pressured and tangential. His eyes dart about as he speaks, and he is unable to maintain eye contact for longer than a few seconds. His attention span is under 1 minute. George appears to have no visual or hearing deficits and in fact seems acutely aware of all the noises and sights around him, as he comments on every sound he hears. He notices every person who walks by the room and bellows out a greeting to them. Several times during the evaluation, he stands up at the table and yells out to someone in the hallway. He is unable to filter out external stimuli during the evaluation. He scores a 4.9 on the Allen Cognitive Disability Levels test.

George appears to have no physical limitations. He ambulates independently with a quick cadence. As he walks, he runs his hands along the walls, possibly to take in more stimuli. The nurses say that he dressed himself this morning, but refused to shower. However, he is clean-shaven. George claims he is independent in all work tasks, but this cannot be verified because he is unable to attend long enough to complete the evaluation.

George responds to questions regarding his leisure time with answers such as, "What leisure time?" and "Leisure is my life!" When asked about attending programs on the unit and being involved with OT, George responds, "I love occupational therapy!" When asked about his goals for OT intervention, his reply is "to make something for the kids in art class."

QUESTIONS

Occupations

1. Identify key ADL occupations in which George has continued to engage and those in which he has not or could not.

2. Identify key IADL occupations in which George has continued to engage and those in which he has not or could not.

3. Identify key sleep–rest occupations in which George has continued to engage and those in which he has not or could not.

4. Identify key work occupations in which George has continued to engage and those in which he could not.

5. Identify key leisure occupations in which George has continued to engage and those he has not or could not.

6. Identify key social participation occupations in which George has continued to engage and those in which he has not or could not.

7. How would you prioritize your OT intervention according to George's occupational needs? Explain your thinking.

Performance Patterns

8. What roles and routines have been disrupted by George's manic episode? How has his engagement in occupation been affected by these disruptions in roles and routines?

9. Describe why it is important for George's occupational therapist to understand his roles and routines.

10. How will this information assist in your intervention planning? Explain your thinking.

Performance Skills

11. Identify 10 key performance skills that are negatively affected by George's current manic episode.

12. Identify 10 key performance skills that are strengths.

13. Are any of the key performance skills you identified as his strengths and barriers the same? If so, explain; if not, could some be categorized as both strengths and barriers?

14. What are some social interaction skills George is currently unable to demonstrate?

15. How would you address George's work issues? What performance skills do you feel are most affecting his work?

Client Factors

16. Identify important values and beliefs that may influence your OT assessment and intervention.

17. Identify 10 key body functions that are negatively affecting George's engagement in occupations.

18. Identify 10 key body functions that are supporting George's engagement in occupations.

19. How would you address George's cognitive issues?

Contexts and Environment

20. Identify key personal and temporal contexts to consider for assessment and intervention.

21. What do you see as social barriers for George? Do they involve his family situation? Can you identify potential supports that are not family members?

22. What are some safety issues that may arise while George is on the unit?

23. What can OT clinicians do to minimize these safety risks during OT groups?

24. How could the treatment team involve George's family in his recovery?

25. At what point in his recovery do you think George would benefit from education regarding his disease?

26. What impact has George's bipolar disorder had on his relationship with his family?

27. How has George's illness affected his relationships at work?

28. How would you interact with the rest of the treatment team?

Theory and Evidence

29. What theory/theories or frame(s) of reference might you use in developing an intervention plan? Describe the rationale for your choice(s).

30. What, if any, evidence can you find to support your choice of theory/theories and/or frame(s) of reference?

31. What, if any, evidence can you find to support intervention?

Intervention Plan and Goals

32. Review again the evaluation session with George. What could have been done to minimize his symptoms and further the evaluation process?

33. Identify assessments that would assist you in completing your evaluation. Why did you choose them?

34. Write a list of some long-term and short-term goals for OT intervention for George.

35. What difficulties would you anticipate while working with George toward his goals?

36. What types of groups do you feel George would benefit from? Why?

37. How could you collaborate with other team members to assist in meeting these goals?

38. What types of groups would be unsafe for George at this time?

39. Write a specific intervention plan, including frequency, for George's 1-week hospital stay.

Situations

40. You invite George to a group, and he agrees to attend. However, he arrives at the group 15 minutes late. George insists you allow him in because you invited him. What would you do?

41. George tells you it is his son's birthday and asks you to allow him to use the staff phone to call home. He tells you that he asked the unit manager, and she said it was all right. You can see that George is anxious and shaking. What would you do?

42. You are in a group with George, and he begins singing aloud. Some of the other patients do not seem to be bothered, but the one sitting next to him gets up and moves her seat. What would you do?

43. George requests that a singing group be held on the unit. The other patient with manic symptoms agrees that she would like to go to a group like that. What are your immediate thoughts about this idea? What would your response be?

44. George signs himself up for a walk to the store with the community living skills group. George does not have privileges to leave the unit at this time. How could you involve George without him leaving the unit?

45. George seems to feel comfortable with you. He asks you if he can call you after he is discharged. How would you respond? How would this make you feel?

Discharge Planning

46. George is being discharged from the hospital. What changes might you expect in his behavior by the time he is ready for discharge?

47. George's wife decides that she does not want him to return to their house after discharge. Do you think he is able to go home and live on his own? If not, what type of placement options would there be for him in the community?

48. George is to attend a day hospital program on discharge from the inpatient facility. What would you expect the OT focus to be in that setting? What recommendations would you make for his OT intervention?

49. Write a discharge note for George.

24

Harold: Polysubstance Abuse

OCCUPATIONAL PROFILE

Harold is a 35-year-old White man who was admitted to the inpatient psychiatric unit of the Veteran's Administration hospital from the emergency department. He was brought into the emergency department by police after getting into a fight at a local bar. Harold was treated for minor cuts and abrasions. The owner of the bar knows Harold well and did not want to press charges.

Harold has a history of alcohol and heroin abuse that goes back 10 years. He started using drugs when he was in Afghanistan and became addicted to heroin and then cocaine. He had been living in his own home and renting out rooms to his friends, but recently lost his home because he was not able to pay the mortgage and is now homeless. He has not been able to hold a job for more than a few months because of his substance abuse. Harold has tried a variety of jobs and has been through several work retraining programs. He found that he likes working with computers; however, he was unable to retain any job in the highly competitive job market. He would end up getting drunk or high and neglect to show up for work for a few days, or to call in.

Harold finished college before enlisting in the Army. His father and grandfather were in the military, and he felt it was his duty to serve as well. Harold was married for 6 years, and he and his ex-wife have one son. They divorced because of his substance abuse problem, and his ex-wife and son moved away; she did not want their son to be influenced by Harold. He has not seen his son since they moved away. Harold has two siblings, but has little contact with either of them. His parents have health issues of their own and live several states away. Harold has tried multiple times to quit drugs and alcohol, but he cannot stay clean and loses his job each time.

Harold would rather have fun than be responsible. He is easily influenced by his friends to go out drinking or do cocaine. His entire social circle is made up of people with whom he either drinks or does cocaine. He cannot make decisions and stick to them because he is easily swayed by others or by the temptation of having fun.

He was admitted to the psychiatric unit for detoxification and discharge planning. Harold would like to get clean, stay clean, get a job, and find a safe place to live. The psychiatrist, occupational therapist, nurse, and social worker on the unit will work with him during his stay. His

Lowenstein NA, Halloran P.
Case Studies Through the Health Care Continuum:
A Workbook for the Occupational Therapy Student, Second Edition (pp 107-109).
© 2015 SLACK Incorporated.

expected length of stay at the Veteran's Administration hospital is 2 weeks.

ANALYSIS OF OCCUPATIONAL PERFORMANCE

At the OT evaluation, Harold presents as disheveled in appearance. He does not have any clothes with him, so he is wearing a hospital gown, hospital robe, and slippers. He is unshaven, his hair is still matted with blood, and it is clear that he has not yet showered. When asked by the occupational therapist if he wishes to take some time to clean up before the interview, he asks, "What's the point?" He is administered an interest inventory and indicates interest in watching sports on TV and going to movies. Harold appears easily distracted, loses his train of thought easily, and needs to ask for questions to be repeated. When given a simple copying task, he has difficulty following directions. He cannot remember the events leading up to his hospitalization. When asked what a typical day was like, Harold cannot give any specific information. He says that he and his buddies just "kinda hang around all day and do whatever we feel like doing."

Harold had to leave the OT evaluation before it was completed because he became anxious and started to shake. It is unclear whether he is truly invested in his recovery process.

QUESTIONS

Occupations

1. Identify two key occupations that you feel Harold should address during his acute hospital stay. Why did you choose these areas?

2. What occupations do you feel Harold is still able to participate in, despite his substance abuse and homelessness? Why?

3. Prioritize a list of occupations that you might address during his hospital stay. Why did you choose these?

Performance Patterns

4. How would you describe a typical day for Harold before his hospitalization? Was this a productive use of his time?

5. What routines have been disrupted by Harold's substance abuse?

6. What roles have been disrupted by his substance abuse?

7. Do you think Harold can return to having productive routines and meaningful roles? Explain your thinking.

Performance Skills

8. Harold does not have any clothing in the hospital and does not seem to care about his appearance. He has not taken a shower or shaved in a few days. How could you address this issue with Harold? What would be the first task that you would try to have Harold work on, and why did you choose this task?

9. Harold has agreed to take a shower, but wants you to be there when he does it. How would you respond to this situation?

10. How would you assess Harold's skills at money management?

11. Harold claims he likes computers, but he has not been able to keep a job because of his substance abuse. What are some of the skills that he needs to be a productive worker? How should OT address these?

12. Harold has limited leisure interests as expressed in his interest checklist. How would you categorize his stated interests, and how would the two of you explore expanding his interests?

13. What social skills can you identify that are supports for Harold? What social skills could assist Harold if he could develop them? How would you assist him in the area of social skills?

Client Factors

14. Identify important values and beliefs that could influence your OT assessment and intervention?

15. Harold has poor time management skills, problem solving skills, and memory. What types of group activities might be beneficial for him?

16. How would you structure tasks so that Harold could follow them?

17. Patients on the unit are responsible for getting to their assigned groups. However, despite having a written schedule, Harold always forgets his groups. How could you address this issue?

Contexts and Environment

18. Identify key personal and temporal contexts to consider for assessment and intervention.

19. What social supports can you identify for Harold? Can you identify new supports? How are his "buddies" as a support system? How would you approach this with Harold and the team?

20. What is the role of OT in educating Harold about his disease? In what ways can OT assist Harold in coping with his disease?

21. Are there programs to assist homeless veterans in your area? Would you refer Harold to them?

22. What other supports does the VA system have for veterans with mental health issues? Would you recommend Harold to any of these? Why or why not?

Theory and Evidence

23. What theory/theories or frame(s) of reference might you use in developing an intervention plan? Describe the rationale for your choice(s).

24. What, if any, evidence can you find to support your choice of theory/theories and/or frame(s) of reference?

25. What, if any, evidence can you find to support intervention?

Intervention Plan and Goals

26. How would you go about completing the OT evaluation?

27. Are there any other assessments that you would like to administer to assist in your intervention planning? What are these, and why did you choose them?

28. How would you engage Harold in identifying some goals for OT?

29. Harold does not understand what OT is and tells you he does not want another "job shrink." How would you explain OT's role in the psychiatric setting?

30. What are some long- and short-term goals for Harold?

31. What obstacles do you anticipate Harold might have in achieving these goals?

Situations

32. One day, when Harold is in group, you think you smell alcohol on his breath. You know that one of his friends visited him earlier in the day. Would you confront Harold? If so, how would you do this, and what might his response be? If not, why not?

33. If you choose not to confront Harold in the situation described in Question 32, what impact might this have on the way you interact with him in your OT sessions?

34. Harold is in one of your groups. He is disruptive, has a short attention span, and keeps talking out of turn. How would you handle this situation?

Discharge Planning

35. What type of setting do you think Harold would benefit from when he is discharged from the VA hospital? Why did you pick this setting?

36. Do you think Harold will need continued OT when he leaves the VA hospital? What do you think he should work on in OT?

37. What would you do if Harold refuses to be discharged to any supportive services, but insists on returning to the homeless shelter?

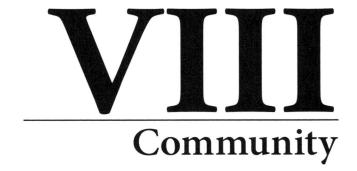

VIII
Community

Gina: Major Depressive Disorder and Alcohol Abuse

Susan Gelfman, MS, OTR/L

OCCUPATIONAL PROFILE

Gina is a 45-year-old, separated White woman with a diagnosis of major depressive disorder and alcohol abuse. She inconsistently attends a partial hospital program. Her history includes multiple suicide attempts and hospitalizations: first at the breakup of a serious relationship in her 30s, another when her mother died of breast cancer 6 years ago, and one when her oldest son went off to college. Her most recent overdose occurred when her husband said he wanted a divorce and moved out of the house. When she left a message on his voicemail, telling him of the overdose, he called 911. She was hospitalized in the acute care hospital for 8 days and then transitioned to the partial hospital program. Gina has worked in a medical office for the past 4 years and had been taking classes at a local community college to become a medical technologist and was doing well. However, for the past two semesters, she has not taken any classes. Gina is a regular churchgoer and used to go to the gym twice a week. She reports having limited social contacts outside her family. She and a female friend sometimes go out for coffee or to a movie. She has a sister, 3 years older, who lives 2 hours away, whom she used to speak with several times a week and visit at least once a month. Recently, she has not been in touch with either her sister or her friend. She also used to help out with children's events at her Catholic church. She used to enjoy watching television reality shows, but even those have not engaged her lately. Gina says her goals for her partial hospitalization are to have help managing her finances, finding an apartment, and returning to work. She was referred to OT for assistance in getting back to work.

ANALYSIS OF OCCUPATIONAL PERFORMANCE

Gina presented to the OT interview with clean hair in need of a cut, poorly fitting clothes, and nails with chipped-polish. She spoke very softly, made poor eye contact, and answered questions briefly. When talking about her family, she became tearful and blamed herself for the divorce. More detailed family information was gathered from the social worker and hospital discharge notes.

According to the social worker, Gina's marriage began to deteriorate when her son left for college 3 years ago. She began to drink three to four cocktails a day, a practice she

Lowenstein NA, Halloran P.
Case Studies Through the Health Care Continuum:
A Workbook for the Occupational Therapy Student, Second Edition (pp 113-115).
© 2015 SLACK Incorporated.

has continued. Her husband responded alternately with withdrawal and verbal abuse. Her children have reacted to the impending divorce in different ways. Her son, Matthew, a college junior, blames his mother. Her daughter, Laura, a freshman in college, has been struggling with depression herself and is on academic probation.

In regard to work, Gina is worried that her last performance review was not good. Her boss cited her frequent absences and her trouble dealing with any problems related to clients.

Gina reports that she has not gone to the gym for a few months because she does not have the energy and becomes easily fatigued. She feels weak and complains of a lack of stamina. She feels guilty about her failure as a wife and mother. She says the rosary daily and frequently goes to confession. She reports that it is hard to concentrate on television or reading now.

When administered the Kohlman Evaluation of Living Skills (KELS; Kohlman-Thomson, 1992), Gina was independent in the following areas: all aspects of safety and health, all aspects of transportation and telephone, purchasing items, obtaining and maintaining a source of income, payment of bills, use of banking forms and plans for employment. She scored needs assist with leisure activity involvement, budgeting monthly income, and budgeting money for food.

Gina completed a Role Checklist (Oakley, 1986). Her current roles include home maintainer, religious participant, and pet owner. Additional past roles are the following: worker, volunteer, student, caregiver, friend, and family member. In the future, she would like to keep her current roles and return to the roles of worker, student, friend, and family member. She identified worker, religious participant, and pet owner as very valuable roles. Friend, student, and family member were somewhat valuable roles.

When tested with the Allen Cognitive Level Screen (ACLS-5; Allen et al., 2007), Gina scored a 5.2. She was able to complete three single cordovan stitches correctly after two demonstrations. Her movements were quite slow. Although she verbalized feeling inadequate to complete the task, she was able to discover successful strategies to correct errors and replicate the corrected stitches.

A home visit was completed. Gina lives alone in a house in the suburbs, which she will need to sell soon as part of the divorce settlement. The house was sparsely furnished as her husband took half of the furniture. The home is in need of repair with leaky faucets, cracked windows, and broken fixtures. There was little food in the refrigerator except for a few frozen dinners. Counters were clean, but dishes were in the sink. The bathroom cabinet had bottles of outdated, unused medications. The living room and dining room were cluttered with stacks of unopened mail and unpaid bills. The bed was unmade, but clean laundry was in the basket. The cat's food and water bowls were filled, and the cat appeared well cared for.

In observations in the partial hospital milieu, Gina missed 1 to 2 days a week, but attends all groups on the days she comes. She says she sleeps poorly, and it is hard to get up in the morning. She stays to herself and does not initiate conversation with other clients. In groups, she responds only when called on.

On discharge, Gina plans to continue with the outpatient therapist she has been seeing for the past 6 months and is willing to continue on antidepressant medications for the time being. She would like to complete her day program within 1 month.

QUESTIONS

Occupation

1. Identify the key occupations that are affected by Gina's depression.

2. What are Gina's occupational strengths?

3. Are there other instrumental ADL issues that could be assessed further?

Performance Patterns

4. In what roles might Gina meaningfully engage in the future?

5. Gina's religious values are both a source of strength and a source of increased guilt. How could positive spirituality be integrated into her intervention?

6. What routines have been most affected by Gina's depression? In what ways have they been disrupted?

7. How can OT make an impact on her performance patterns?

Performance Skills

8. Identify 10 performance skills that negatively affect Gina's occupational performance.

9. Identify 10 performance skills that may be supports in her occupational performance.

10. What is the status of Gina's social relationships?

Client Factors

11. What neuromuscular factors might hinder Gina's attainment of her goals? How could these factors be addressed?

12. Which groups could address performance skill problems in emotion regulation, cognition, and communication?

Contexts and Environment

13. What safety risks exist with Gina's unused medications?

14. Are there ways Gina can strengthen her support network at the day program? At home?

15. Gina's sporadic attendance at the day program decreases her access to treatment and has a negative impact on her insurance payment. How could you address this issue with her? How could you, as a therapist, encourage Gina's increased participation in the milieu?

16. Would you involve Gina's family in education about depression? If so, which family members would you include, and which symptoms of depression would you focus on?

17. Given Gina's occupational profile and her ACLS-5 score of 5.2, what supports would you predict she will need in the community?

Theory and Evidence

18. What theory/theories or frame(s) of reference might you use in developing an intervention plan? Describe the rationale for your choices.

19. What, if any, evidence can you find to support your choice of theory/theories and/or frame(s) of reference?

20. What, if any, evidence can you find to support intervention?

Intervention Plan and Goals

21. Are there other assessments that could provide additional information about Gina's overall occupational profile?

22. What assessment(s) could be used to further evaluate her medication management skills?

23. What are your hypotheses regarding Gina's occupational functioning from the KELS, ACLS-5, and Role Checklist? How would you incorporate these into your intervention planning?

24. Write a list of short- and long-term objectives for Gina based on her stated goals.

25. What, if any, obstacles do you see to Gina reaching her goals?

26. Describe how education about depression could help Gina with her feelings of guilt.

Situations

27. Gina is crying in the hall just before group. She has just received a verbally abusive phone call from her husband. What would you do?

28. Gina reveals to the morning check-in group that her daughter did not come over the weekend as promised. Gina says, "She'll be really sorry after I'm gone." What would you do?

29. Gina reports in the weekend planning group that she plans to go out to a bar with her sister on Saturday night. What should you do?

30. Gina has looked at a few apartments, but there is nothing in her price range that she will accept. It is time for her to leave the program. What community resources for clients with mental illness could continue to help her with this goal?

Discharge Planning

31. Would you refer Gina to any professional- or peer-led support groups in the community? If so, which ones?

32. Gina has been coming to groups regularly. Her attention and her decision-making and problem-solving skills have improved. She would like to return to work and wants to call her boss. How could you assist her in planning this encounter? What concerns might her boss have about Gina's return to work?

REFERENCES

Allen, C. K., Austin, S. L., David, S. K., Earhart, C. A., McCraith, D. B., & Riska-Williams, L. (2007). *Allen Cognitive Level Screen—5 (ACLS–5)/Large Allen Cognitive Level Screen—5 (LACLS–5)*. Camarillo, CA: ACLS and LACLS Committee.

Kohlman-Thomson, L. (1992). *Kohlman Evaluation of Living Skills*. Bethesda, MD: The American Occupational Therapy Association.

Irene: Posttraumatic Stress Disorder

OCCUPATIONAL PROFILE

Irene is a 19-year-old Latina woman with a diagnosis of posttraumatic stress disorder (PTSD). She has a secondary diagnosis of loss of peripheral vision in her left eye, which resulted from a childhood playground accident. She has no other diagnoses. Irene has been attending a partial hospitalization program for several months due to PTSD after a fire in her home 14 months ago took the lives of her mother and two young brothers. Irene was not at home at the time of the fire. She had been called in to work to fill in for another employee. Irene works as an assistant manager for a large pharmacy chain that has stores open 24 hours. Upon leaving the store after midnight, Irene went out for pizza and then drove home. She drove down her street around 1:30 a.m. to see "smoke and flames everywhere!" Her house was engulfed in flames.

Irene's PTSD has interfered with all aspects of her life. Before the fire, she had worked full time at the store, but she has not been to work since the accident. Irene had also been enrolled part time in a bachelor's degree program with the intent of receiving her degree in business management. Irene is a sophomore, but she has not attended classes since the fire. Before the fire, she was outgoing; loved to go out dancing on the weekends; and enjoyed movies, cooking, and shopping with her friends. She enjoyed school and was looking forward to a professional career. Since the fire, Irene has stopped spending time with her friends and chooses to spend most of her time alone. She speaks very little and avoids interaction with others.

Irene is currently living with her aunt and uncle. Her Aunt Marlene is her mother's sister. Marlene has told Irene she can stay indefinitely. There is plenty of room in the house because all of Marlene and Douglas's children have grown and moved away. Since she moved in with her aunt and uncle, Irene has been attending church weekly with them. Irene's father, who lives out of state, has said she could move in with him, but Irene has declined. Her goals are to return to school, finish her degree, and "not feel so bad all the time."

ANALYSIS OF OCCUPATIONAL PERFORMANCE

Irene was evaluated by OT using interview, chart review, Role Checklist, and observation. She is cooperative and

Lowenstein NA, Halloran P.
Case Studies Through the Health Care Continuum:
A Workbook for the Occupational Therapy Student, Second Edition (pp 117-119).
© 2015 SLACK Incorporated.

quiet. She compensates easily for her loss of left peripheral vision. Functionally, she has difficulty concentrating, which affects her short-term memory and immediate recall. She has a slightly delayed reaction when responding to open-ended questions, but quickly answers yes/no questions. Irene does not initiate conversation nor does she ask any questions. On the Role Checklist (Oakley, 1986), Irene identified the following past roles: student, worker, doing things with her family, doing things with friends, and church. The only role she could identify as "currently doing" was "doing things with her family." When asked to explain why she put this as both a past and present role, she noted that her past family included her mother and siblings and her current family is her aunt and uncle. She noted the roles that she "would like to do" as student, worker, doing things with friends, and church. She identified all of these roles as "very important." Irene has persistently been experiencing thoughts of the tragedy both in dreams and while awake. She frequently reports "reliving" the experience at the sight or suggestion of fire. She reports physiologic reactivity such as sweating and shortness of breath whenever there is any reminder of the accident. Irene has also been experiencing symptoms of depression, insomnia, decreased concentration, and frequent crying episodes, followed by emotional numbness. She appears tired and lacks energy. Irene is independent in her self-care. She is neat and well groomed, wearing a simple sweat suit and sneakers. "At least I can still do that for myself," she says. Irene reports no leisure activities or hobbies at this time. Irene cries several times during the evaluation even though she is asked no questions about the event or her family.

QUESTIONS

Occupations

1. Identify occupations that have been negatively affected by Irene's PTSD in the area of ADLs, work, education, social participation, and leisure.

2. How would you prioritize these for intervention? Did you consider Irene's goals when prioritizing these occupations?

3. In what occupations is Irene still actively engaged?

Performance Patterns

4. How does the information from the Roles Checklist assist you in your understanding of Irene's engagement in occupation?

5. How would you use this information for intervention planning?

6. Which of Irene's routines have been disrupted?

7. How has the disruption in Irene's routines affected her engagement in occupations? Is this an area that OT could address in the partial hospitalization program? If so, how? Do you feel it would be useful to address this disruption in routines?

Performance Skills

8. Identify 10 key performance skills that are supporting Irene's current engagement in occupations.

9. Identify 10 key performance skills that are negatively affecting her engagement in occupations.

10. What could be done in the partial hospitalization milieu to increase Irene's social interactions with others?

11. What could be done to increase Irene's social interaction with her friends?

12. What performance skills are having the greatest impact on Irene's work and social interaction occupations?

13. Can you describe an intervention session to address these performance skills?

Client Factors

14. Identify important values and beliefs that could influence your OT intervention.

15. How might positive spirituality be integrated into Irene's intervention?

16. Identify the key body functions that are impeding Irene's engagement in occupation.

17. Identify the key body functions that are supporting her engagement in occupation.

18. Describe how the cognitive deficits Irene is experiencing are affecting her on a daily basis. Do these also have an impact on her routines? If so, how?

19. What day-to-day difficulties would you anticipate Irene would have given these cognitive deficits?

20. Would you expect these deficits to be temporary or permanent? Explain.

Contexts and Environment

21. Identify key personal and temporal contexts to consider for assessment and intervention.

22. Are there cultural contexts to consider? What are these?

23. What type of education would Irene's aunt and uncle benefit from to help Irene engage in her desired occupations of work, school, and social interaction?

24. Can you incorporate the virtual context into your intervention? If so, in what way would you do this?

Theory and Evidence

25. What theory/theories or frame(s) of reference might you use in developing an intervention plan? Describe the rationale for your choice(s).

26. What, if any, evidence can you find to support your choice of theory/theories and/or frame(s) of reference?

27. What, if any, evidence can you find to support intervention?

Intervention Plan and Goals

28. What goals would you and Irene set for her OT intervention?

29. What are Irene's strengths?

30. How could Irene capitalize on her strengths to help her meet her goals?

31. Write an OT intervention plan for Irene, including frequency of attendance. In which OT groups would you recommend Irene participate?

Situations

32. Irene has not attended any groups except the community meeting each morning. She tells you she does not want to go because she is sure she will begin crying for "no reason." What would you say?

33. Irene's case manager asks if you could work with her around her job skills. How could you incorporate Irene's job tasks into your intervention?

34. Irene is in the day room with a new patient. The new patient asks Irene why she is there, and Irene's response is "because I'm crazy." How could you respond to Irene's answer? Why might Irene have responded like that?

35. Irene tells you that she got a call from one of her coworkers, which she did not take. She says she does not know how she can face them. How would you respond?

36. You are sitting with Irene and she asks you, "Have you ever lost anyone?" What would you say?

Discharge Planning

37. Irene is to be discharged from the partial hospitalization program. She will be seeing a psychologist weekly for counseling and monitoring of medication adherence. She will not be receiving any other services, including OT. How could you help Irene to carry over what she has learned from OT?

REFERENCE

Oakley, F. (1984). The role checklist. National Institute of Health, Department of Rehabilitation Medicine, Occupational Therapy Service. Washington, DC: U.S. Government Printing Office.

27

Leo: Schizoaffective Disorder

OCCUPATIONAL PROFILE

Leo is a 31-year-old Black man with a diagnosis of schizoaffective disorder. His first episode was when he was 24 years old. Leo also has a secondary diagnosis of cannabis abuse. He is attending the partial hospitalization program to assist in his transition from the acute care hospital back to the community and his job. Leo was hospitalized for a little more than 3 weeks with symptoms of auditory hallucinations, withdrawal and isolation, hypersomnia, and psychomotor retardation. Leo's hallucinations disappeared, but he still exhibits the other symptoms—though to a lesser degree.

Leo lives in a group home with four other men with chronic mental illness. Leo has been living there for several years and gets along well with his housemates. Leo's parents are divorced. His father has schizophrenia and is occasionally found wandering and sleeping on the streets. Although he is not homeless, Leo's father often leaves his rooming house, and is picked up later by the police for sleeping on other people's property. Leo's mother drinks heavily and regularly. She lets Leo visit her at the house when she is sober. Otherwise, she threatens him and kicks him out. Leo

has one sibling, a sister, who is not involved with the family in any way.

Leo does well at the group home. He is independent in his ADLs, with occasional reminders, and he participates in the chores around the house. Leo is responsible for setting and clearing the table and taking out the trash weekly. He does his own laundry when he runs out of clean clothes. He spends most days hanging out in the common room of the home playing video games, watching television, or shopping online, or else sleeping in his room. He states, "I like being alone." When he was in high school, he was on the basketball team and was used to working out with his teammates. He has not been physically active since his graduation from high school. He smokes two packs of cigarettes a day.

Before his hospitalization, Leo worked approximately 8 to 10 hours a week with a cleaning company that contracts to clean offices at night. The supervisor picked Leo up on Tuesday nights at 9 p.m. and drove him and another employee to the one or two locations that needed service that night. The men worked until the jobs were finished, and the supervisor drove Leo home. Many Tuesdays, the supervisor had to wake Leo up to get him to work, but

Lowenstein NA, Halloran P.
Case Studies Through the Health Care Continuum:
A Workbook for the Occupational Therapy Student, Second Edition (pp 121-124).
© 2015 SLACK Incorporated.

Leo never refused to go. He has had this job for the past 8 months and appears committed to keeping it. His supervisor, Scott, feels that, even though Leo works slowly, he is a good employee and more reliable than most.

Leo's goals are to return to his job, and he would like to go to school to learn a trade. He will attend the day program 5 full days a week.

ANALYSIS OF OCCUPATIONAL PERFORMANCE

Upon admission, Leo was evaluated through chart review, information from the hospital discharge note, the social work intake, interview, and observation during a group activity. During the evaluation, Leo presented as withdrawn and minimally interactive. He was appropriately groomed and dressed. He did speak when spoken to, but answered in one- or two-word sentences. There was a delayed response when he answered, and his speech was slow and labored. He rarely made eye contact and stared down at his shoes throughout most of the evaluation.

During the group activity, Leo exhibited decreased problem solving, short-term memory deficits, and decreased attention span. Moreover, his working memory was poor. He also showed decreased organizational skills. He does not have any apparent sensory or perceptual deficits.

Leo's posture is slightly kyphotic, his hips in a posterior tilt, and he shuffles a bit when he ambulates. His ambulation is slow, but he has no balance problems. His AROM and strength are within functional limits, but his coordination is slow and dexterity is impaired bilaterally. Leo says, "I feel stiff. I can't move right," when asked to perform simple manual tasks. He reports doing his own self-care and nods yes when asked if it takes longer than it used to. He shakes his head no when asked if he has resumed his chores at the group home. Leo states that he has no pain.

Leo has had multiple hospitalizations because of his schizoaffective disorder. Sometimes stressors in his life precipitate his hospitalizations, and other times he simply stops taking his medications. Occasionally, the onset of the acute symptoms of his illness do not appear linked to any factor at all. This is one of those times.

Leo was admitted to the hospital at the request of his case manager after several weeks of auditory hallucinations, which included voices talking about him negatively, sirens, and loud music. Leo became depressed when the voices spoke badly of him and began to sleep more, eat less, and grow increasingly isolative. The staff from the group home noticed his behavior changes and notified Leo's case manager, who, in turn, called his psychiatrist. Leo's doctor recommended his admission to the acute care hospital.

Leo's case manager, Amelda, has been working with him for 7 years. Leo trusts both her and his psychiatrist, Dr. Ramkasoon, and rarely disagrees with what either of them recommend. Leo does not like to go to the hospital, but he dislikes the auditory hallucinations even more. He was discharged into the day program. He has been to this program in the past.

Leo agrees to participate fully in the schedule at the day program. He is concerned about it interfering with his appointments with Dr. Ramkasoon and is reassured that those appointments take precedence over the groups at the day program. Leo has participated in OT in the past and is vaguely familiar with its purpose.

QUESTIONS

Occupations

1. Identify the occupations in which Leo is currently engaging. Would any of these occupations be addressed in OT?

2. Identify the occupations that Leo's recent hospitalization has disrupted. Would any of these occupations be addressed in OT?

3. Which of the occupations you have identified need to be addressed immediately and those that can be addressed in a few weeks. Explain your thinking. Did you consider Leo's goals when prioritizing the occupations?

4. In your opinion, does Leo have adequate leisure activities in his life? Explain your answer.

Performance Patterns

5. How have Leo's routines been disrupted by the recent exacerbation of his illness and his hospitalization?

6. Would you administer any assessments to learn more about his routines?

7. What type of adaptations to Leo's daily routine might make it easier for him to accomplish tasks in less time?

8. What type of adaptations might be necessary to Leo's work routine? What could his supervisor reasonably be expected to accommodate?

9. What roles have been disrupted by Leo's recent illness and hospitalization?

10. Would you address this role disruption? If so, how? Would you administer any assessments to learn more about his roles?

Performance Skills

11. Identify 10 key performance skills that support Leo's engagement in occupation.

12. How might you structure intervention for Leo to be able to perform his ADL with greater ease and speed? How could you assess whether this intervention is working?

13. Describe an intervention to address three of the performance skills using activity and occupation intervention methods.

14. How would you assess whether this intervention has an effective outcome?

Client Factors

15. Identify important values and beliefs that may influence your OT intervention?

16. Identify 10 key body functions that are strengths for Leo.

17. Identify 10 key body functions that are impairing his daily functioning.

18. How are Leo's cognitive issues affecting his engagement in occupations?

19. How would you assess his cognitive status more thoroughly? Which assessment(s) would you use and why?

20. What evidence is there to support the use of this assessment or these assessments for individuals with schizoaffective disorder?

21. What types of activities might be difficult for Leo given his motor deficits?

22. What specifically would you recommend to deal with Leo's dexterity and coordination deficits?

23. How could you ensure carryover of these recommendations for Leo when he is not at the program?

Contexts and Environments

24. Identify key personal and temporal contexts to consider for assessment and intervention.

25. Are there any environmental adaptations that could be useful for aiding Leo in engaging in his roles, routines, and occupations?

26. What might be some safety concerns during Leo's attendance at the day program?

27. What type of precautions could the staff take to ensure Leo's safety while he is participating in the day program? At the group home?

28. How might Leo explain to his supervisor why he has missed so much work?

Theory and Evidence

29. What theory/theories or frame(s) of reference might you use in developing an intervention plan? Describe the rationale for your choice(s).

30. What, if any, evidence can you find to support your choice of theory/theories and/or frame(s) of reference?

31. What, if any, evidence can you find to support intervention?

Intervention Plan and Goals

32. Are there additional assessments that you would like to administer to gain more information? If so, what are they, and why did you choose these particular assessments? Do they address engagement in occupation or specific performance skills or specific client factors?

33. What specific goals for OT would you help Leo set for himself?

34. What goals would you set for OT intervention?

35. How do your goals and the ones Leo might have differ?

36. How might Leo utilize his strengths to achieve his goals?

37. Identify groups from which you feel Leo would benefit.

38. What methods of intervention should be used for Leo to meet his goal of returning to work?

Situations

39. Leo's psychiatrist, Dr. Ramkasoon, asks you to write up a protocol about how you assess work readiness so that he may better understand the process for future patients. Write an outline of the protocol you would give him.

40. You are helping Leo review his schedule for the week. He cannot follow it and appears to "shut down" when presented with too much information at once. How can you present Leo's schedule to him in a manner that he can understand?

41. To help prepare for resuming chores at his home, Leo agrees to clear the table after lunch in your program. After his first day, you notice he has forgotten several empty glasses on the table. Why might this have happened? How could you use this opportunity to assess Leo's skills? How would you use this information in your next session with Leo?

42. The director at the group home calls asking for some exercises for Leo to do at home so he will not be so "zombie-like." However, Leo tells you he does not like exercise anymore and will not do them. What activities can you suggest that would incorporate movement

into Leo's daily routine so that he does not feel like he is exercising?

43. Leo's supervisor, Scott, calls the day program wondering how Leo is doing and when he will be back at work. What are you allowed to tell Scott, according to Health Insurance Portability and Accountability Act (HIPAA)? What would you say?

Discharge Planning

44. From an OT perspective, what objective information would tell you when Leo is ready to leave the day program?

45. What supports would you want to make sure are in place before discharge?

Henry: Primary Care Health and Wellness Intervention

OCCUPATIONAL PROFILE

Henry is a 53-year-old man who has a history of type II diabetes mellitus and obesity. He has smoked since he was 14 years old. He is divorced and lives alone in a second-floor walk-up apartment. He works full time in information technology for a large biomedical company. His job requires long hours at a computer. Because he has no one at home, he usually takes on the projects that will require long hours and often leaves work after 9 p.m., after having started work at 8 a.m. He enjoys his job and coworkers.

Henry has one grown son who is married and lives a 3-hour plane ride away. They speak on the phone, but Henry does not often visit. Henry enjoys reading the daily newspaper and books, but spends most of his time online even on weekends.

Henry had a recent visit to his primary care provider (PCP), who was very concerned about his diabetes and weight. Henry's diabetes has been poorly controlled because his diet is mostly fast food or frozen meals. He has tried to stop smoking and to lose weight in the past, but his attempts have always failed. Henry has gone on many diets and has joined many gyms, but he has difficulty sticking to any diet or exercise program.

Henry's physician has referred him to the occupational therapist in his office for a health and wellness intervention. His insurance will pay for eight OT visits.

ANALYSIS OF OCCUPATIONAL PERFORMANCE

Henry arrives 30 minutes late to his appointment with you, stating that he had to complete part of a project before he could leave work. He is asked if he understands why his PCP has referred him to OT and whether he understands what OT is about. He notes that he is not sure what to expect from his visit. Henry reports that he does not believe that he can lose weight. He slowly started gaining weight in his thirties, as his marriage became more stressful and he was pursuing a master's degree in computer science. Between the long school hours, his job, and the stress of his relationship, he started eating more junk food and drinking sodas and caffeinated drinks to stay awake; he also began missing meals. He smokes about a pack and a half a day, and because he cannot smoke in the office, he has to go outside to smoke. His boss does not mind this because Henry often

Lowenstein NA, Halloran P.
Case Studies Through the Health Care Continuum:
A Workbook for the Occupational Therapy Student, Second Edition (pp 125-127).
© 2015 SLACK Incorporated.

works late, and his work is excellent. After his divorce, he stopped caring about cooking or what he ate and continued to gain weight. He is now 67 pounds above his ideal body weight. Henry lists all of the many diets his can remember having tried, including low carb, high protein, Weight Watchers ("too many women," he says). He feels that his work schedule makes it difficult to stay on any diet, and he admits that he does not know how to cook anything aside from eggs, pasta, and fried chicken.

Henry was diagnosed with type II diabetes 5 years ago and he has been on insulin injections for 4 years. He readily admits that he does not monitor his blood sugar very well, but he does not see this as a problem. He figures that it all works out over the course of a week. When asked, he does mention that he has some numbness in his fingers and assumes this is from all the computer work that he does. He says that he would love to lose weight, but lacks confidence that his lifestyle will enable this to happen.

QUESTIONS

Occupations

1. Identify which of Henry's occupations you would like to learn more about. Why?

2. How would the information from Question 1 assist you in developing an intervention plan for Henry?

3. What would you see as Henry's current occupations?

4. How would you explain to Henry the role of OT in a health and wellness context?

5. Look at the occupations listed in the *OTPF* and identify occupations that you might explore with Henry. Why did you choose these?

6. Are there occupations that you feel would be beneficial for Henry to explore? Why?

Performance Patterns

7. How do Henry's routines and roles contribute to his health and wellness?

8. What do you see as the biggest barrier to Henry being successful in changing his habits and routines?

9. How many roles does Henry identify that he currently engages in? Do you see any past roles that he has given up?

10. How might the identification of Henry's roles be helpful in developing an intervention plan for him?

Performance Skills

11. Identify 5 to 10 performance skills that you feel are Henry's strengths.

12. Of the 5 to 10 performance skills identified in Question 11, which ones would you use during your intervention?

13. In which category do most of the performance skills identified in Questions 11 and 12 fall? How would the understanding of these performance skills assist you in developing a health and wellness intervention for Henry?

Client Factors

14. What are some of Henry's beliefs, and how might they influence your intervention?

15. What are some of Henry's values, and how do these differ from his beliefs?

16. How might his values influence your intervention?

17. The *OTPF* describes the client factor of spirituality. Explain this concept and how you see it applying to Henry's OT wellness intervention.

Contexts and Environment

18. Identify how the cultural, temporal, personal, and virtual contexts are contributing to Henry's current lifestyle.

19. How might you influence these contexts to support Henry's ability to change his health behaviors?

20. Describe the social supports and barriers in Henry's environment. How would these influence your OT intervention?

21. Describe the physical supports and barriers in Henry's environment. How would these influence your OT intervention?

Theory and Evidence

22. What theory/theories or frame(s) of reference might you use in developing an intervention plan? Describe the rationale for your choices.

23. What, if any, evidence can you find to support your choice of theory/theories and/or frame(s) of reference?

24. What, if any, evidence can you find to support intervention?

Intervention Plan and Goals

25. How would you go about developing goals for Henry's health and wellness intervention?

26. What assessments would you want to complete that would assist you and Henry in identifying goals for OT intervention?

27. How would you document to obtain payment for Henry's intervention? What aspects of intervention would you emphasize and why?

28. Knowing that you only have eight visits with Henry, what would be the frequency of your OT intervention sessions? Why?

29. Describe what you would expect to cover in your eight intervention sessions.

30. What theoretical framework(s) would you use for your OT intervention? Explain your thinking.

31. What evidence is there to support the use of OT in a health and wellness context? For diabetes education and management? For weight loss?

Situations

32. During your first intervention session, Henry is very negative and notes he does not see why his PCP has sent him to see OT. He has tried to lose weight and stop smoking in the past, but he cannot keep with any program. How do you respond to this?

33. Henry comes to his OT appointment and has not done the homework that you asked him to do. This homework was to keep a daily activity log for 2 weekdays and 1 weekend day. He says it is too much trouble and he does not know how it will be useful. How would you respond?

34. Henry reports that he was able to meet with a nutritionist and develop a nutrition plan. He kept to it for 1 week and tells you it was too hard to manage. He understands that it is important to eat better, but does not know how to make this a regular habit. How would you help Henry?

35. You have seen Henry for six of his eight appointments. He had been coming to his appointments on time and completing most of his homework; however, he is now 20 minutes late, and the PCP's receptionist tells you that he just called and wants to cancel his final two appointments. What would you do?

Discharge Planning

36. Henry has completed all eight of his appointments. He has been managing his nutrition well, with occasional lapses. He expresses to you that he is not sure that he can maintain this without your support. You will not be paid for any further OT visits. What other supports might you explore with Henry so that he can continue to make gains?

37. Are there other professionals you would suggest as referrals for Henry?

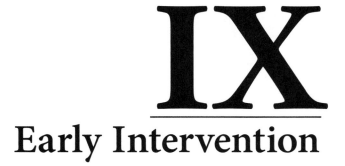

IX
Early Intervention

Joey: Early Intervention—
Delayed Developmental Milestones

Debra G. Sharp, MEd

OCCUPATIONAL PROFILE

Joey is a 24-month-old boy. He was born on a U.S. Navy Base in Guam. He lives at home with both of his parents and his two older brothers, aged 5 and 7 years. Joey's dad is in the U.S. Navy. They recently moved from Guam to San Diego, California. The move was a difficult adjustment for the entire family as it involved a new city, new schools, new friends, and new jobs. They have received a lot of family support, and temporary housing from the Navy. Now that Joey's brothers are in school and adjusting to their routines, Joey's mother has started participating in local Mommy and Me baby groups once a week. Joey's mother reported that he has always been different from her other two boys. He seemed to develop slower. He was a colicky baby and has never eaten or slept well. He was just "different." Now that life has "calmed down" and Joey is having play dates with other 2 year olds, his mother is seeing a big difference. Joey prefers to be alone and does not even appear to notice anyone else in the room. When another child comes near him, he will not interact with him or her, but will grab the toy he is playing with and not let go. He does not seem very excited when his brothers or father come home from school. He appears to recognize them all, but does not get excited for them or anyone else. His mother reports a normal pregnancy with Joey and he was born at 38 weeks. She breastfed him and he would nurse for 20 to 30 minutes every 3 hours. He cried a lot, even after feeding, and he always appeared to be hungry. Joey was not putting on weight, so the pediatrician supplemented his feedings with formula, and he slowly started to put on weight. As an infant, Joey never slept more than 30 minutes at a time. His mother reports that he never seemed to hit the developmental milestones other babies did. She reported that, with her husband working on the Navy ship for the first 6 months of Joey's life, she "was barely surviving." All she wanted was for Joey to eat, gain weight, and sleep. She could not handle more than that. She decided to contact her new pediatrician. The pediatrician told her to go for a free developmental screening. Joey's mother is hoping to find out if there is anything wrong with Joey and to have him be a happy boy, like his brothers.

Lowenstein NA, Halloran P.
Case Studies Through the Health Care Continuum:
A Workbook for the Occupational Therapy Student, Second Edition (pp 131-133).
© 2015 SLACK Incorporated.

ANALYSIS OF OCCUPATIONAL PERFORMANCE

Developmental Screening: At the time of the screening, Joey is 24-months-old. He is screened using the Hawaii Early Learning Profile (HELP; Teaford, Wheat, & Baker, 2010) in the areas of cognitive, language, fine motor, and gross motor skills, and social and emotional development. Joey can pull himself to standing and can walk along furniture. Mom reports that he can walk independently, but prefers to crawl because it is faster. He uses pincer grasp to pick up tiny objects, bangs two cubes together, and puts toys into a container. Screams and cries comprise most of his language, although he does say a few one-word utterances: "mama," "no," "up," "na-na" (this last designating water). Joey does not make eye contact with the person talking. If he wants something, he points and screams. His mother said she has tried using baby sign language with him, but he just screams. He is beginning to imitate the sign for "more" and "eat." When she finally figures out what he wants, she gives it to him immediately. He does not follow simple one-step directions and appears to be ignoring whoever is making the request. When looking at a book, he hits the picture when named. He likes to shake, throw, and drop new objects. When songs are sung, he moves his body to the music, claps his hands, and smiles. His mother reports that he does that at home as well. Joey wears a diaper and shows no sign of being uncomfortable in it. He does not dress himself. He will hold his arms up to assist in dressing and undressing. When he wants to go outside, he grabs his coat and bangs on the outside door. He eats mostly pureed baby food; his mother reports that he chokes when she feeds him thicker food. He does not attempt to feed himself, but will hold the spoon; however, his mother feeds him every meal and snack. His mother says that he has been sleeping 8 hours at night with one 2-hour nap during the day.

QUESTIONS

Occupations

1. In what age-appropriate occupations would you expect Joey to be engaging?

2. In what occupations do you feel Joey and his mom are currently engaging?

3. In what occupations do you feel Joey and his mom should be engaging?

4. Are there issues with the occupations in which Joey is currently engaging?

Performance Patterns

5. Who are your clients for this intervention? How would you include them in your teaching?

6. Discuss the routines that Joey's mother has in terms of taking care of Joey. Are these helpful routines? Explain your thinking.

7. Describe what you think a typical day for Joey's mom might be like. Is this a well-balanced routine? Why or why not?

8. What roles does Joey's mom fulfill? How do you hypothesize she is feeling about these roles? With which one(s) do you feel OT might be able to help her? Explain your thinking.

Performance Skills

9. Identify key performance skills that are supports for Joey's engagement in occupation.

10. Identify key performance skills that are barriers to Joey's engagement in occupation.

11. Describe an intervention that addresses some of these performance skills.

12. What toys or games would you use during intervention sessions to address these performance skills?

Client Factors

13. Identify important values and beliefs that may influence your OT intervention.

14. Identify 10 key body functions that are strengths for Joey's engagement in occupation.

15. Identify 10 key body functions that are barriers to Joey's engagement in occupation.

16. What toys or games would you use during intervention sessions to address these body functions?

Contexts and Environment

17. Identify key personal and temporal contexts to consider for assessment and intervention.

18. Are there cultural contexts to consider as you assess and plan your intervention? If so, what are they, and how might they influence your assessment and intervention?

19. Given the information that you have, how might you adapt or change Joey's home environment to encourage social interaction with his family?

20. How would you incorporate Joey's brothers into your intervention sessions in his home? At the Early Intervention Center?

21. What information would you provide to Joey's parents regarding his behaviors and engagement in occupations? Explain your thinking.

Theory and Evidence

22. What theory/theories or frame(s) of reference might you use in developing an intervention plan? Explain the rationale for your choice(s).

23. What, if any, evidence can you find to support your choice of theory/theories and/or frame(s) of reference?

24. What, if any, evidence can you find to support intervention?

Intervention Plan and Goals

25. Identify the major issues that should be addressed by OT. Explain why you chose these.

26. Are there other assessments that you would like to administer? What are they, and why did you choose them?

27. Write an individualized family service plan for Joey.

28. From what other disciplines do you feel Joey would benefit from receiving services? Why?

Situations

29. You are in a session with Joey and his mother in their home when Joey's mom suddenly bursts into tears and says, "I can't take this anymore. I just want a normal son!" How do you respond?

30. Joey's 5-year-old brother is trying to engage him in a game involving rolling a ball to each other on the floor and looking at each other. His brother stops playing and says he does not want to play anymore because Joey is no fun to play with. He would rather play with his other brother. How would you explain Joey's behavior to his brother?

31. Joey's mother and father take you aside as you are leaving their home after one of their sessions and ask you to be truthful with them. They then ask you whether Joey will ever be "normal" and want to know what is wrong with him. What would you tell them?

32. One day in a play group in the Early Intervention Center, you see Joey engage in play with another child for a few minutes. How would you respond to this? Would you try to engage him in social play again? Explain your thinking.

Discharge Planning

33. When would you start discussing the transition out of early intervention into preschool with Joey's parents?

34. Who else would be involved in the transition discussion?

REFERENCE

Teaford, P., Wheat, J., & Baker, T. (2010). *HELP 3-6 assessment manual* (2nd ed.). Palo Alto, CA: VORT Corporation.

Brynn: Preschool—
Delayed Developmental Milestones

Debra G. Sharp, MEd

OCCUPATIONAL PROFILE

Brynn is a 48-month-old girl who lives at home with her mother, father, 6-year-old sister, and 24-month-old brother. Both parents work outside the home. All three children have been attending child care centers and/or school since the age of 3 months. According to her parents, Brynn gets along well with her siblings and enjoys playing dressup and watching Sesame Street and other children's shows. She loves to swing on the playground, but her mother reports that she will not go near the sandbox and often refuses to wear long-sleeved shirts or "itchy" sweaters. Brynn's parents reported that there have been "red flags" in Brynn's development, but they just assumed she would eventually "catch up." The family recently moved, and her new preschool teacher had a meeting with her parents sharing her concerns about Brynn's development. After the meeting, the parents contacted their pediatrician and asked for an early childhood assessment referral from the local school system.

ANALYSIS OF OCCUPATIONAL PERFORMANCE

Brynn was assessed using the following standardized assessments: The Learning Accomplishment Profile—Diagnostic Version (Chapel Hill Training Outreach Project, Inc., 2005) for fine motor, cognitive, and language skills; Ages & Stages 54-Month Parent Questionnaire (Squires & Bricker, 2009) for gross motor skills and self-help and task-related skills; Battelle Developmental Inventory (BDI-2; Newborg, 2004) for social/personal interaction skills; clinical observation; and interview with her mother and preschool teacher.

Behavioral Observations: Standardized testing took place in an empty classroom in the preschool and occurred over two sessions. The first session lasted approximately 45 minutes. Brynn was cooperative and attempted all items presented to her. After approximately 20 minutes, Brynn wanted to play and repeatedly asked, "I pay?" as she would

Lowenstein NA, Halloran P.
*Case Studies Through the Health Care Continuum:
A Workbook for the Occupational Therapy Student, Second Edition* (pp 135-138).
© 2015 SLACK Incorporated.

complete tasks. Each time, she was easily redirected back to the task at hand. On three separate occasions, when patted on the back or touched on the arm for praise, Brynn would pull her body away, turn her head away, and cover her eyes. Several times, Brynn had difficulty making eye contact while listening to directions for testing items. She became more comfortable as testing continued.

The second testing session lasted approximately 30 minutes. Although Brynn willingly completed tasks, she frequently needed to be prompted to speak louder, to wait (she attempted to turn the pages of the stimulus book quickly), and to focus on testing items. When administering the speech portion of the assessment, Brynn needed to be asked to repeat herself because her volume was often low and she would not directly face you. Attempts to reposition Brynn were unsuccessful in that Brynn would twist her body so that she was not looking directly at you. Eye contact during the second testing session was limited. The results are considered to be an accurate reflection of Brynn's abilities.

Fine Motor: Brynn was unable to string small and large beads because she would not push the beads down on the string. She built a tower of 10 small blocks and wove a string randomly through holes in a sewing board. She put pegs in a pegboard and built two steps with three small blocks when shown a model. She cut with scissors after a demonstration, but used an inappropriate hand grasp (thumb down). She was not able to build a bridge with large blocks from a model. Brynn holds pencils with a two-finger fisted grasp up high on the pencil. She was able to imitate vertical and horizontal lines, circular strokes, intersecting lines (cross), and the letter H. She copied a circle, but was not able to imitate the letter V, trace a diamond, or draw a person with two parts (she drew a cross and said it was "mommy").

Cognitive: Brynn matched eight color cards and independently named each color to include orange, red, green, yellow, brown, purple, blue, and black. She matched simple shapes, pictures of like objects, and pictures of like animals (and identified the animals). Brynn did not receive credit for matching complex objects (6 of 10) nor did she receive credit for completing a six-piece inset puzzle of a cow in 3 minutes (she placed 3 of 6 pieces). Brynn was unable to form a square from two triangles to match a design. She identified the "big" and "little" blocks on request two times each. She responded to the concepts of "empty" and "full" and the prepositions "over" and "under." She placed "only one" block on request and pointed to the group with "more" two times. Brynn rote counted "1 to 5, 10" and counted blocks to 3 ("one, do, dee"). She was unable to rote count or count objects to 10.

Language: Brynn's total language score indicates that her language skills are delayed. Strengths were noted in naming colors, naming the missing part in pictures, and pointing to numerals. Limitations were exhibited in naming the cause of events ("what makes water boil?"), naming

three activities recently performed, selecting pictures that match a verbal description, and responding appropriately to prepositions. According to an interview with Brynn's teacher from part-day preschool, Brynn demonstrates inadequate functional communication abilities. Strengths were noted in nonverbal behaviors, including the use of facial expressions, use of gestures, and following a teacher's nonverbal communication (i.e., finger raised to lip to be quiet). Limitations were found in conversational routines and skills, and in asking for and giving information. Brynn's skills are emerging in waving or saying hello or goodbye, demonstrating turn-taking rules during play and in the classroom, and maintaining attention while another person is speaking. Brynn does not yet demonstrate the following skills on a consistent basis: looking at the person to whom she is speaking; initiating conversation with friends; joining games or conversations; communicating verbally when playing with children; introducing new topics of conversation; asking for help from others; asking for permission to play with a friend; asking questions if she is confused; offering to help others; or telling the details of an experience or story.

Personal/Social: The results from this area are obtained through teacher report on the BDI-2 from Brynn's preschool teacher. The personal/social domain measures those abilities and characteristics that allow the child to engage in meaningful social interactions. The behaviors measured are grouped into three subdomains: adult interaction, peer interaction, and self-concept and social role. Brynn demonstrates strengths in her adult interaction skills. Her skills have recently emerged into initiating interactions with familiar adults and using adults other than parents as resources. She follows adult directions with little or no resistance, imitates the play activities of other children, shows sympathy and concern for others, shares property with others, states her first name, uses objects in make-believe play, and uses her name to refer to herself. Brynn exhibits limitations in her peer interaction and in her self-concept and social role skills, most specifically as they involve using verbal communication in a social manner. Brynn demonstrates parallel play, but is not yet showing cooperative play skills. She is reluctant to engage in new or unexpected activities. Brynn does not yet initiate social or verbal interactions with peers.

Gross Motor: Brynn's mother reports that Brynn hops on one foot without losing her balance and throws a ball overhand toward another person. She states that Brynn can jump forward a distance of 20 inches from a standing position and is beginning to be able to catch a ball with both hands from a distance of 5 feet. Her mother also reports that Brynn can balance on one foot for at least 5 seconds and can walk on her tiptoes for 15 feet. Brynn scored 55 of 60 possible points. Gross motor development is within normal limits according to this screening tool per parent report.

Adaptive/Self-Help: Brynn scored 30 of 30 possible points on the adaptive domain of the Ages & Stages 54-Month Parent Questionnaire. Brynn's mother reports that Brynn can wash and dry her hands independently. She also reports that Brynn brushes her teeth independently by putting toothpaste on the toothbrush and brushing all of her teeth without help. Her mother notes that Brynn can serve herself food using large utensils, and she was observed eating and drinking without difficulties.

Relationship of Findings to Educational Functioning: Results from assessments show that Brynn is developing at age level in the areas of gross motor and adaptive skills; however, there are significant delays in the areas of cognitive, fine motor, communication, and social skills. Delayed developmental skills could adversely affect Brynn's participation in typical preschool activities.

QUESTIONS

Occupation

1. Identify the primary occupations that Brynn's assessments demonstrate may be impaired for her age.

2. Identify the primary occupations that Brynn's assessments demonstrate may be typical for her age.

3. Explain your thinking for your responses to Questions 1 and 2.

4. Prioritize the occupations to work on in OT from most important to least important. Explain your reasoning for these priorities.

Performance Patterns

5. Are there performance patterns that are important to consider during your OT intervention?

6. What issues regarding performance skills might you want to explore further with Brynn's parents?

7. Do you consider Brynn's parents to be your clients? Explain your answer.

8. Do you consider Brynn's siblings to be your clients? Explain your answer.

Performance Skills

9. Identify 10 key performance skills that are supports for Brynn's engagement in occupations.

10. Identify 10 key performance skills that are barriers to Brynn's engagement in occupations.

11. Describe an activity that would address some of these performance skills during intervention.

12. How would you explain the importance of these performance skills with the rest of the early intervention staff?

Client Factors

13. When thinking about the "client," what values and beliefs should you consider in developing your intervention plan? Why?

14. Identify 10 key body functions that are strengths for Brynn.

15. Identify 10 key body functions that are barriers to Brynn's development.

16. Describe an intervention to address some of the body function deficits. Be specific in describing how the activities address the client factors you identified.

17. Using Brynn's assessment data, how would you prioritize your intervention? Explain your thinking.

Contexts and Environment

18. Identify key personal and temporal contexts to consider for assessment and intervention.

19. Are there cultural considerations? If so, what are they?

20. Describe how you would communicate with Brynn's preschool teacher so that she will carry over your goals in the preschool.

21. Describe how you would communicate with Brynn's parents so that they will carry over your goals in the home.

22. Would you recommend any adaptations to Brynn's home or preschool environment? If so, describe them and explain how you would expect the preschool staff and/or Brynn's family to support her engagement in occupation in the chosen setting.

Theory and Evidence

23. What theory/theories or frame(s) of reference might you use in developing an intervention plan? Describe the rationale for your choice(s).

24. What, if any, evidence can you find to support your choice of theory/theories and/or frame(s) of reference?

25. What, if any, evidence can you find to support intervention?

Intervention Plan and Goals

26. Write a list of the functional problems that OT might address for Brynn and her family.

27. Are there one or more specific OT assessments that you would like to administer? Explain which assessment(s)

you would choose and why you feel this would assist in your development of a comprehensive individualized education plan (IEP).

28. Write a list of goals for Brynn's IEP and describe how these relate to preschool activities.

29. Describe an intervention session during the play group that you run in the preschool with the speech-language pathologist. Would you be working on the same goals or different goals?

30. Describe some of the activities, games, and toys that you would use during your interventions with Brynn.

Situations

31. You and the speech therapist are running a play group in the preschool. The children are sitting in a circle, singing songs and playing instruments. Suddenly, Brynn starts yelling and pulling at her top and trying to take it off. What would you do?

32. During a home visit, Brynn's older sister is playing a game with dolls with you and Brynn. Brynn's sister starts to "spank" her doll very hard and yells at her that she is not behaving. Brynn immediately runs away and cowers in the corner of the room. How do you respond to this situation? Explain your reasoning.

33. You are observing in Brynn's preschool and notice that Brynn's teacher is making Brynn do finger painting. You can see that Brynn is uncomfortable and resisting, but the teacher keeps insisting that Brynn make a "painting for mommy, like all the other children are doing." After a few minutes, Brynn bursts into tears and runs over to you. Explain what you would do.

34. You have determined that Brynn has some sensory integration issues of tactile defensiveness. You have given Brynn's mother a routine to do twice a day to help desensitize Brynn. After a few weeks, you have noticed no change and ask Brynn's mother about this. She tells you that she has enough on her plate with taking care of three children, working, and managing their home. You feel this is an important area to address for Brynn. What would you do and why?

Discharge Planning

35. Brynn is going to be transitioned to kindergarten in 1 year. Transitions are difficult for Brynn. When do you start preparing for this transition, and how do you make sure it is a smooth transition for Brynn and her family?

REFERENCES

Chapel Hill Training Outreach Project, Inc. (2005). *Learning Accomplishment Profile—Diagnostic Version (LAP-D) (3rd edition): Examiner's manual & technical report.* Lewisville, NC: Kaplan Early Learning Company.

Newborg, J. (2004). *Battelle Developmental Inventory* (2nd ed). Boston: Houghton Mifflin Harcourt.

Squires, J., & Bricker, D. (2009). *Ages & Stages Parent Questionnaires: A parent-completed monitoring system* (3rd ed.). Baltimore: Brooks.

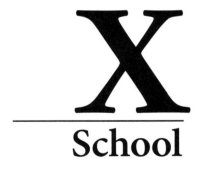

X
School

31

Maggie: Leukomalacia

Cathie Marqusee, MS, OTR/L

OCCUPATIONAL PROFILE

Maggie is a 6-year-old girl who lives at home with her parents and 4-year-old sister. She is in the first grade at an inner-city public school. Her father is a firefighter, and her mother is a stay-at-home mom who regularly volunteers at Maggie's school while Maggie's sister is at preschool. Maggie has diagnoses of leukomalacia and mild cerebral palsy with significant spasticity in the LEs and mild spasticity and weakness in her left UE. She has a complicated medical history, beginning at birth. She was born prematurely (29 weeks), weighing 2 lbs 8 oz. She had hernia surgery at 4 months and underwent surgery for congenital hip dysplasia at 14 months. Early intervention services began at that time, with a primary focus on PT for mobility. OT services began in preschool.

Maggie is a hard worker who is highly motivated to learn and to keep up with her peers. She has strong cognitive abilities and a wealth of knowledge about the world around her. She loves school, enjoys social interactions with both adults and peers, and is well liked by all. She enjoys reading, loves animals, and often talks about the pet cat she has at home. She also enjoys being active and particularly loves dancing and singing in music class. Although she is willing to engage in a wide variety of activities in school, play with peers is at times affected by her physical challenges, and she requires close supervision for safety on the playground.

Maggie strives to be independent and is persistent with even the most challenging tasks. She is, however, aware of her challenges, gets frustrated at times, and reports that her peers often comment on her inability to write legibly or draw pictures with recognizable people or objects. Also, while Maggie is close to her younger sister, she has recently become aware of the fact that her sister's fine motor skills have surpassed hers.

Maggie's mother is extremely dedicated to her children and does her best to expose them to a variety of cultural and recreational activities outside of school. Like Maggie herself, she is determined not to let Maggie's physical challenges keep her from doing everything her peers are doing. Because of this, Maggie occasionally finds herself in unsafe situations, and she has had a number of falls recently. Maggie wants desperately to keep up with her peers in the community and gets frustrated when she is unable to do so. Her mother has been encouraged to have Maggie use her posterior walker for added stability when she is in a crowd

Lowenstein NA, Halloran P.
Case Studies Through the Health Care Continuum:
A Workbook for the Occupational Therapy Student, Second Edition (pp 141-144).
© 2015 SLACK Incorporated.

where she might be bumped or is walking a long distance, but she is resistant to doing so. She is so happy that Maggie no longer needs the walker at all times like she used to, and feels that using it would be regressive and would cause her to appear more disabled than she is.

Maggie currently receives OT services at school to address significant fine motor and visual motor delays, as well as difficulty with visual tracking and visual perception. She also receives PT services to address poor strength and endurance in her LEs. It is hoped that, given continued OT intervention and classroom accommodations, Maggie will be able to get her thoughts down on paper effectively and will attain basic fine motor skills for writing, drawing, coloring, using scissors, fastening her clothing, and throwing and catching a ball.

ANALYSIS OF OCCUPATIONAL PERFORMANCE

A recent OT reevaluation was administered using the visual motor and fine motor subtests of the Miller Function and Participation Scales (M-FUN; Miller, 2006). This assessment uses workbook and play activities to assess a child's functional performance related to school participation. The test items are motivating and playful, and include such early school activities as writing, drawing, tracing, cutting, and object manipulation. The Beery-Buktenica Developmental Test of Visual-Motor Integration (VMI; Beery, Buktenica, & Beery, 2010) was also administered to gain additional information about Maggie's ability to integrate visual perception and motor coordination as she copied a variety of shapes and designs. Clinical observations related to postural, visual, and other sensorimotor skills were also considered, as was a report from the classroom teacher. During testing, Maggie consistently demonstrated the ability to follow directions and sustain attention to a task without difficulty. Maggie's scores on the M-FUN were as follows: visual motor scaled score—2; fine motor scaled score—1 (the mean scaled score on the M-FUN is 10, and the average range is 7–13). Her standard score on the VMI was 61 (the mean standard score on the VMI is 100, with an average range of 90–110). Decreased proximal stability, as well as mild muscle tightness and weakness throughout her UEs, especially on her left side, affect Maggie's seated posture and effective use of her arms and hands for fine motor and visual motor tasks. She tends to bend over the table with her head close to her work, and her posture is rarely symmetrical.

Maggie is right-hand dominant and attempts to stabilize and assist with her left hand, although this is somewhat challenging for her, especially when cutting with scissors. She grasps her pencil and markers with a three-finger grasp, with all fingers extended and a narrow web space. Her wrists are often in a flexion position, rather than in a more efficient extension position. Poor hand strength was evident as she manipulated clay on the M-FUN; she was unable to use enough force to form a ball or a snake with the clay. Maggie also has difficulty manipulating fasteners, such as buttons and zippers, on her clothing and pouring liquids without spilling. She is able to use a fork and spoon successfully when eating. She is also able to use a functional pincer grasp to pick up small items.

On the M-FUN, Maggie had great difficulty staying between the lines on simple maze activities. When cutting a fish shape, she had difficulty with accuracy (straying up to a half-inch from the line), and the cuts were choppy, leaving ragged edges. She is able to trace upper case letters well, but has great difficulty copying letters legibly because the lines are wobbly and the orientation is often skewed, with the letters sometimes lying on their side. Letters that contain diagonal lines are particularly challenging. When asked to draw a person, most body parts are included, although they are often hard to recognize because of difficulties with line control and proportion and orientation of the parts. For example, the legs often emerge from the side of the head, and the eyes are drawn too large to stay within the boundaries of the head.

On the VMI, Maggie was able to successfully copy simple shapes, such as vertical and horizontal lines and a circle. She was unable to correctly copy diagonal lines, a square, a triangle, or an X.

Although Maggie is able to make and maintain eye contact, she has great difficulty visually tracking moving objects and has mild difficulty with convergence and divergence. With the help of occasional Botox (Allergen, Inc.) treatments to decrease spasticity and orthotics to support her ankles, she is able to maneuver well throughout the school environment as long as she takes her time. She requires close supervision on stairways because she tends to rush and could easily get bumped by a peer, which would cause her to lose her balance. Also, the assistive technology specialist has recently provided Maggie with a portable word processor with text-to-speech and word prediction to support her writing in the classroom.

In the classroom, Maggie has great difficulty writing, coloring, and drawing at a level commensurate with her peers. She also has great difficulty controlling scissors and catching or throwing a ball. Given accommodations for written output, she is on grade level with all academics and is reading above grade level.

QUESTIONS

Occupations

1. Identify occupations in which Maggie continues to participate.

2. Identify the occupations that are difficult for Maggie.

3. Given Maggie's age, identify occupations in which she should be, but is not, able to participate.

4. Given Maggie's disability, name four ADLs that she might have difficulty with in the school environment.

Performance Patterns

5. Who are your clients? How does this influence your intervention?

6. Identify current roles that Maggie fulfills. Are these appropriate for a child her age? Explain.

7. Can you identify age-appropriate roles that Maggie is not currently participating in? Explain why you chose these.

8. What routines would you help Maggie's mother establish? Explain why you feel these are important routines to develop.

Performance Skills

9. Given that Maggie struggles so much with handwriting and she is beginning to use a word processor, do you think there a reason to continue working on handwriting with her? Please explain.

10. Would it be realistic to expect Maggie to draw a recognizable picture of a person with 8 to 10 well-proportioned parts connected correctly within the next year?

11. How might you work with Maggie around drawing a person more effectively? List four activities you might try to this end.

12. How would you help Maggie to color more accurately within the boundaries of a picture?

13. Name four activity ideas that would encourage Maggie to draw diagonal lines.

14. Name four activity ideas to help Maggie to develop increased arm and hand strength.

15. Name four activity ideas to help Maggie develop increased pencil control.

16. What could you do with Maggie before fine motor tasks to decrease spasticity in her arms?

Client Factors

17. Identify important client values and beliefs that could influence your OT intervention.

18. List four activities you could do with Maggie to encourage visual tracking. Can you anticipate the functional ramifications of Maggie's difficulty with visual skills as she moves up the grades in school?

Contexts and Environment

19. Identify key personal and temporal contexts to consider for assessment and intervention.

20. What types of classroom accommodations could be implemented to help Maggie sit upright and symmetrically?

21. What types of classroom accommodations might be implemented to help Maggie maintain a functional tripod grasp with extended wrist, open web space, and thumb–index finger opposition?

22. What could her Maggie's parents do at home to ensure that her sister's skills, relative to hers, do not affect Maggie's self-esteem?

23. How would you work with Maggie's teacher to ensure follow-through?

24. How would you work to educate Maggie's mother regarding the activities in which Maggie can safely participate, when she might be unsafe in the community, and how to make accommodations so that Maggie can safely participate in those activities?

Theory and Evidence

25. What theory/theories or frame(s) of reference might you use in developing an intervention plan? Describe the rationale for your choice(s).

26. What, if any, evidence can you find to support your choice of theory/theories and/or frame(s) of reference?

27. What, if any, evidence can you find to support intervention?

Intervention Plan and Goals

28. Write a handwriting goal for Maggie's new individualized education plan (IEP), keeping in mind that IEP goals are meant to be realistically achievable during the upcoming 1-year period.

29. Write four short-term objectives toward meeting the handwriting goal.

30. Write a goal for scissors skills, both in terms of grasp and accuracy.

31. Write four short-term objectives toward meeting that goal for scissors skills.

32. What observations were made that would indicate the need for more information regarding Maggie's visual perceptual skills?

33. How could you further assess Maggie's visual perceptual skills?

REFERENCES

Beery, K. E., Buktenica, N. A., & Beery, N. A. (2010). *Beery-Buktenica Developmental Test of Visual-Motor Integration (VMI)* (6th ed.). San Antonio, TX: Pearson.

Miller, L. J. (2006). *Miller Function and Participation Scales (M-FUN)*. San Antonio, TX: Pearson.

Jane: Transition From Preschool to Kindergarten

Iris G. Leigh, CAGS, OTR/L

OCCUPATIONAL HISTORY

Jane is a preschool student who will enter kindergarten in September. She was 4.8 years old at the time of referral to OT. She is a very verbal child who enjoys school and has many friends. She is petite for her age and wears her long, dark hair in braids.

Jane attends the Backyard Preschool and Daycare 5 days a week and will begin at Green Elementary School in September. Her mother and teacher have discussed some areas of her development that concern them. Although Jane enjoys many of the activities at school, she does not readily engage in either fine or gross motor tasks unless directed by an adult.

Jane lives with her single mother and younger brother in a second-floor apartment in an urban setting. She has little access to a yard or green spaces that are close to her home. Jane's mother reports that she is too tired and overwhelmed with work and household obligations to take Jane and her brother outside to play after school or on weekends. She states that Jane is obedient and helps her with household chores, especially cooking. Jane knows the names of the neighbors in the other apartments and often visits her elderly neighbor. Jane has cousins who live nearby and she plays well with them. She shares toys and dolls with her family. She also loves to help her mom around the house. Jane and her family use the public library, and she often sits with her brother during story hour at the library.

Although Jane has not been able to independently dress herself or play outside on playground equipment, her mother did not initially identify these as problems. Jane states that she often dresses Jane in the morning so that she will not be late for school. She brushes and braids her hair every morning. She feels this is an intimate time for them to talk and enjoy each other's company. She is pleased that Jane is beginning to read. She is not as worried about her difficulties writing and manipulating fine motor materials.

In school, Jane is well behaved, listens to adults, shares, and takes turns in play activities. She enjoys socializing with other children, plays with dolls, and claps her hands in rhythm to music. Jane loves to sing and look at books. She can identify the letters in her name and is beginning to sound out simple three-letter words. The school staff felt that Jane was immature and was falling behind on activities that were heavily based on fine and/or gross motor skills. As the school year moved closer to the expectations

Lowenstein NA, Halloran P.
*Case Studies Through the Health Care Continuum:
A Workbook for the Occupational Therapy Student, Second Edition* (pp 145-147).
© 2015 SLACK Incorporated.

for kindergarten, both Jane's mother and the teachers at the Backyard Preschool and Daycare became apprehensive that Jane was not making sufficient progress in these areas. Jane expressed frustration and/or avoidance with motor activities. Both Jane and her mother would like her to become more competent and confident in her abilities to complete the functional tasks expected for entry to kindergarten. Jane was referred by her preschool teacher for an OT evaluation because of a suspected delay in her fine and gross motor skills.

Analysis of Occupational Performance

In addition to seeing the OT, it was recommended that Jane be assessed by a team of school professionals. The team members who evaluated Jane included the classroom teacher, school psychologist, OT practitioner, special education teacher, and the adaptive physical education teacher. Adults and children are so drawn to Jane's strong social and verbal skills that they often do not notice that she avoids many other school tasks that are important to her learning.

The OT administered selected subtests of the Hawaii Early Learning Profile (HELP; Teaford, Wheat, & Baker, 2010) to assess her overall occupational performance in school. Gross motor skills were below expected levels. Jane was unable to balance on either foot independently, kick a ball rolled directly to her, or alternate feet when descending steps. She backed away when a ball was gently thrown to her and was unable to pedal a tricycle. Overall strength and ROM appeared within expected limits, except in the areas of trunk and hand strength. Some minor weakness was noted in these areas. On the HELP assessment, Jane was also delayed in her fine motor skills. She was unable to string large beads or cut with a scissors. Her ability to draw was also limited. She could draw a circle, but was unable to draw a representational figure with features that that were recognizable.

The OT observed Jane in the classroom and on the playground. For small group sessions, Jane sat at the classroom table leaning with her head in her hands. Bilaterally, she was able to hold down her paper with one hand and scribble with her other. She attended well to classroom activities and followed two- to three-step directions. Jane spoke in complete sentences and could verbally identify all of the letters of her name. During free time, she gravitated toward the kitchen and doll areas, socializing with other children. She did not approach the block and building table unless coaxed by an adult. She played dress-up, but often asked the adults or other children for help putting her arms in the sleeves of clothes and buttoning. At the end of the day, Jane was not able to put her coat on independently and needed help zipping it. During a classroom cooking activity, she was observed to roll dough and readily put her hands in the mix.

On the playground, Jane stayed close to the adults. She would sit on a swing, but did not ask to be pushed. She did not join in with games that required her to catch, throw, or kick a ball. When the children ran and chased each other, Jane joined in for brief times, but often ran slowly and awkwardly. If tagged by the other children, she sat on the sidelines and did not ask to rejoin the activity. She did not run efficiently around obstacles on the playground. Jane is reluctant to ascend or descend the slide independently. She has difficulty riding a tricycle, balancing on one foot to play games, and running around obstacles. When children start playing ball games, she sits on the sidelines and talks to the adults.

Jane's mother was interviewed and asked to describe how Jane negotiated self-care activities at home. She reported that Jane washed her hands and assisted in washing her body in the bath. She was completely independent in toileting and in brushing her teeth. Jane's mother felt that Jane was fairly independent in dressing; she said that Jane was able to put on pants and t-shirts, but had more difficulty with other items of clothing, mostly when they were in a hurry or when there were small fasteners. Jane could use a fork and spoon to eat her food. She needed assistance cutting or spreading food with a knife; however, Jane's mother did not give Jane an opportunity to use a knife very often. After completing the evaluation process, the individualized education plan (IEP) team met, and she was diagnosed with a developmental delay. An IEP was developed to address her functional motor and ADL needs.

Questions

Occupation

1. What are the main areas of Jane's occupations that were assessed by the OT?

2. What other areas would you think should be assessed to depict a clearer picture of Jane's strengths and challenges?

3. Do the teacher and parent describe Jane's skills the same way? If not, how do they differ?

Contexts and Environment

4. What are the environmental and client factors that influence what Jane can complete at home and in school?

5. What environmental changes would you implement to decrease Jane's frustration with school tasks?

6. Can you suggest any adaptive equipment that could help Jane better access school activities?

7. What would you say to justify the need for OT services at the IEP meeting?

8. What would you suggest to help OT work with the other professionals on the IEP?

9. What would you consider critical points that would support Jane's and her mother's concerns?

10. Are there any areas of safety that need to be considered when providing intervention services?

Theory and Evidence

11. What theory/theories or frame(s) of reference might you use in developing an intervention plan? Describe the rationale for your choice(s).

12. What, if any, evidence can you find to support your choice of theory/theories and/or frame(s) of reference?

13. What, if any, evidence can you find to support intervention?

Intervention Plan and Goals

14. Given the IEP process, what do you think should be the major long-term and short-term goals for Jane?

15. What accommodations might Jane need to succeed in school?

16. In what other school activities might Jane need adaptations and related services?

17. What interventions would best help Jane access school-wide tasks?

18. What interventions would support Jane's independence with ADL?

19. What information and consultation services to the teacher and other school personnel would support Jane's progress in the classroom?

20. What home programming ideas would you suggest for Jane's mother?

21. What would you implement to best support Jane's desire to accomplish specific tasks and to decrease her overall frustration with fine and gross motor activities?

22. Describe the most effective OT and OT assistant supervision model for Jane's OT program.

23. How would the legal aspects of the Individuals With Disabilities Education Act affect Jane's service delivery?

REFERENCE

Teaford, P., Wheat, J., & Baker, T. (2010). *HELP 3-6 assessment manual* (2nd ed.). Palo Alto, CA: VORT Corporation.

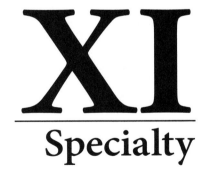

XI
Specialty

33

Gloria: Burns—Superficial, Partial, and Full-Thickness

Occupational Profile

Gloria is a 44-year-old bilingual Latina woman with a diagnosis of burns to 39% of her body. She has superficial burns on 5% of her body, partial-thickness burns on 24% of her body, and full-thickness burns on 10% of her body.

Gloria is a divorced mother of three. She owns her three-bedroom ranch-style house in a small suburb. She works as a chef for a large corporate catering firm. While at work, Gloria had set up the stovetop to begin preparing food for the day's meals. As she turned on the gas, the stovetop exploded into flames, burning Gloria severely. Luckily, she turned her face away quickly enough to avoid severe facial burns or inhalation injury. Gloria was taken immediately to a hospital and transferred to the burn intensive care unit (ICU). She was in the ICU and acute care portion of the hospital for 4 weeks and is being transferred to the rehabilitation hospital for continued intensive therapy. She has skin grafts over her full-thickness burns. The grafts are autografts, taken from her left thigh. Because Gloria was in good health before her accident and a nonsmoker, the doctors feel her partial-thickness burns are likely to heal themselves and have decided against grafting those areas.

The doctors feel she is progressing well and is an excellent candidate for continued rehabilitation.

Gloria is a busy single mother and, between work and her children, she does not have much time for pursuing outside interests. She cannot even remember what her former interests were since it seems it has been such a long time since she could enjoy them. She does try to attend church as often as she can and has been going to the same church for 10 years. She enjoys the community and the pastor. After her divorce, Gloria decided that she needed a profession that would allow her to have a career. She enrolled in a local culinary school and paid for the tuition on her own. She is proud of her accomplishment and feels she demonstrated to her children how to overcome adversity. Gloria's three children (aged 14, 12, and 9) are staying with her sister while she is in Shriner's Hospital. Although the two younger children visit Gloria often, the older one does not like being in the hospital and comes only occasionally.

Gloria's employers have set up a worker's compensation case manager to oversee the treatment and hospital progress. Gloria's brother-in-law wants Gloria to sue to ensure her and her family's financial future. Gloria wants to get better and does not feel she can deal with the additional stress of a legal battle right now. Gloria's sister, Tina, and

Lowenstein NA, Halloran P.
Case Studies Through the Health Care Continuum:
A Workbook for the Occupational Therapy Student, Second Edition (pp 151-154).
© 2015 SLACK Incorporated.

TABLE 33-1

GLORIA'S ACTIVE RANGE OF MOTION

	LEFT UPPER EXTREMITY	RIGHT UPPER EXTREMITY
Elbow flexion	110 degrees	120 degrees
Elbow extension	-10 degrees	-5 degrees
Wrist extension	20 degrees	25 degrees
Wrist flexion	25 degrees	60 degrees
Ulnar and radial deviation	10 degrees	10 degrees
Supination	45 degrees	80 degrees with pain
Pronation	60 degrees	85 degrees with pain
PIP/DIP flexion	45 degrees	55 degrees
MCP flexion	80 degrees	85 degrees
Digit extension	-10 degrees	-5 degrees
MCPs extension	-10 degrees	N/A
MP flexion	20 degrees	25 degrees
IP flexion	10 degrees	15 degrees
Thumb extension	-5 degrees	WNL
Palmar abduction	15 degrees	25 degrees
Radial abduction	Trace	15 degrees
Opposition	Lateral side of third digit	Lateral side of fourth digit

her family have been supportive. Her ex-husband lives out of state and is remarried with his own family. Gloria's sister called to tell him about the accident. He offered no help other than to wish her a quick recovery. Gloria's parents are both living, but are in poor health. They offer to do whatever they can to help. Gloria's pastor is visiting her weekly for prayer. Gloria wants to return home and to start working as soon as she is able. She does not want to be a burden to her family. The plan is for Gloria to remain at the hospital until she is able to care for herself at home and then attend outpatient therapy.

ANALYSIS OF OCCUPATIONAL PERFORMANCE

Gloria is seen for an OT evaluation the day after her hospital admission. "Where have you been?" she asks. "The occupational therapist at the other hospital was in to see me right away. I need to get going to get home. Please help me." Gloria's eyes are sad and her voice is soft. Gloria had suffered burns to her hands, arms, anterior trunk, and neck area. The full-thickness burns are on the dorsum of her hands and posterior forearms. She also has a small area of partial-thickness burns on the forearms. Her trunk has partial-thickness burns, and the left side of her face has only superficial burns. By looking at the location of Gloria's burns, you can see that she turned her head to the right and pulled her arms up to protect her face.

Gloria presents without any cognitive, visual, hearing, or perceptual deficits. She has sensory deficits on the dorsum and webbing of both hands, left side of face, posterior forearms, and anterior trunk related to the burns damaging the dermis. She also has sensory deficits in the left upper-arm area. Her skin in the damaged area is painful in some spots and not in others. The pigment is red and the skin is very taut and dry. Her forearms are covered with "second skin." The chart reveals that there are several "weepy" areas that are not healing well, making Gloria susceptible to infection.

Gloria has AROM within functional limits in her trunk and shoulders. Gloria's AROM is listed in Table 33-1.

Gloria scored below the norm for the Jebsen Hand Function Test.

Gloria is right-hand dominant. Her strength and coordination were not formally assessed, but are obviously impaired because of the severity of her injuries. Gloria says she is frequently in pain and gets relief only from the medications.

Gloria is able to transfer to and from the bed and chair with minimal assistance. She has fallen once in the hospital after attempting to get up too quickly. She needs assistance occasionally to turn in bed because of the pain. She ambulates without a device with contact guard. Gloria complains of pain in the left leg around the grafted area.

Gloria requires total assistance to bathe because of her fragile skin and the need for nursing to check her skin thoroughly and apply medication. She is able to put on her own shoes (Velcro sneakers), loose socks, and sweatpants. She has not been wearing a bra. She is able to put on a pullover shirt with minimal assistance. Gloria can do all of her oral hygiene herself, but usually asks for help because it "never feels clean enough" to her.

Gloria had been responsible for all the household duties and care of her children. She is still unable to perform those duties at this time. Gloria admits to feeling upset about what happened. "God has mysterious plans for us. I just never thought he'd have this in mind for me," she remarks with sorrow.

Gloria agrees to participate in whatever treatment is necessary to get her home. She is to be seen by the physician, nursing, OT, PT, the dietitian, and social worker. She says her goals for herself are to be able to take a shower and to be able to take care of her daughters.

QUESTIONS

Occupation

1. Identify the occupations that have been negatively affected by Gloria's burns.

2. Identify the occupations in which Gloria can continue to engage.

3. What do you think are Gloria's most valued occupations?

Performance Patterns

4. What roles and routines have been most negatively affected by Gloria's current condition?

5. What roles and routines have not been affected by Gloria's current condition?

6. Why is it important to understand Gloria's roles and routines for developing an OT intervention?

Performance Skills

7. Identify 10 performance skills that have been affected by Gloria's condition.

8. Identify 10 performance skills that can be supports during OT intervention.

9. Explain how you would organize an ADL session with Gloria, with the focus on teaching bathing techniques.

10. What precautions would you need to take to ensure Gloria's safety during an ADL retraining session?

11. Write a plan to restore Gloria's AROM. What types of activities would you use? Are they preparatory, purposeful, or occupation-based?

12. How would you address Gloria's hand function (strength and coordination)? Would you use preparatory methods and tasks, activity interventions, or occupation-based interventions?

13. Gloria says she does not feel emotionally ready to be in the OT room near the kitchen area. How would you respond? Who might you tell about this?

14. Before Gloria is ready to begin shower training, what would you have to teach her?

15. What types of purposeful and occupation-based activities could you plan for your interventions?

Client Factors

16. Identify important values and beliefs that could influence your OT intervention.

17. In what way might Gloria's spirituality influence her response to her accident? How might her spirituality aid in the rehabilitation process?

18. What are the physical complications that could develop following severe burns? Explain in detail.

19. What are the precautions that should be taken to promote burn healing?

20. What are the signs of hypertrophic scarring?

21. What OT techniques can be used to prevent scar formation?

22. Gloria asks you to explain the scarring process to her. Write out what you would tell her.

23. Gloria tells you she feels like her clothes are "itching" her, and it is irritating for her to have anything touch her skin. Why might this be? How would you explain it to Gloria? What can Gloria do to get relief from the itching?

24. Write out a protocol for intervention focusing on desensitization.

25. How would you assess Gloria's strength and coordination on an ongoing basis?

Contexts and Environment

26. Identify key personal and temporal contexts to consider for assessment and intervention.

27. Identify social supports that could be important for Gloria during her recovery. How can OT assist in engaging these supports?

28. What type of adaptive equipment might Gloria need to begin regaining independence in daily tasks?

29. What are the pros and cons of issuing adaptive equipment to a person in burn rehabilitation?

30. What type of emotional impact do you think this injury has had on Gloria? On her family?

Theory and Evidence

31. What theory/theories or frame(s) of reference would you use in developing an intervention plan? Describe the rationale for your choice(s).

32. What, if any, evidence can you find to support your choice of theory/theories and/or frame(s) of reference?

33. What, if any, evidence can you find to support intervention?

Intervention Plan and Goals

34. Develop a list of problems that may be addressed by OT during Gloria's rehabilitation stay. How would you prioritize this list? Why did you prioritize it as you did? How would you take Gloria's wishes into account?

35. Are there other assessments that you would consider using in developing an intervention plan? What are these, and why did you choose them?

36. What are Gloria's strengths and what are the barriers she may encounter?

37. What long-term goals would you and Gloria set for her OT intervention?

38. What short-term goals would you help Gloria set for herself in regard to OT intervention?

39. Using the OTPF, what approaches would you use during your interventions? Why?

Situations

40. You are performing PROM with Gloria, and she is in obvious pain. She tells you to keep going. Would you? Why or why not?

41. You are teaching Gloria how to care for her night hand splints. She tells you they hurt and the night nurse takes them off for her. This was the first you had heard of this. What would you do?

42. The weekend occupational therapist scheduled to see Gloria reports that she refused Sunday treatment. When you ask Gloria, she says it is a day of rest and reflection. She asks not to be scheduled by OT or PT on Sundays. What do you think is more important, therapy or religion, and why?

43. Gloria's burns are healing well, and she is now able to perform her bathing with only minimal assistance. She wants to go home for the holiday weekend and stay at the home of her sister, Tina, overnight. Tina has agreed to assist her with ADLs. What education should you give Tina before Gloria goes on the leave of absence?

44. Gloria is still not feeling ready to begin any meal preparation tasks. Her daughters have offered to do the hot meal preparation at home. Should you continue to try to work toward independence in meal preparation using only the microwave? Why or why not?

Discharge Planning

45. Gloria's discharge plans are to return home and attend outpatient OT. What do you feel should be the goal of outpatient therapy?

46. Upon discharge, Gloria and her doctor ask you if you think she can drive now. What factors must be considered? What would you say?

47. Write a home OT program for Gloria.

REFERENCE

Jebsen, R. H., Taylor, N., Treischmann, R. B., Trotter, M. J., & Howard, L. A. (1969). An objective and standardized test of hand function. *Archives of Physical Medicine and Rehabilitation, 50(6),* 311–319.

34

Violet: Right Flexor Tendon Laceration, Depression

OCCUPATIONAL HISTORY

Violet is a 31-year-old White woman with a diagnosis of a right wrist flexor tendon laceration following a suicide attempt. Violet also has a diagnosis of depression. She had never attempted suicide before. Violet, or "Vi" as she prefers to be called, was referred to outpatient OT by her hand surgeon.

Vi had become distraught after her parents threatened to "disown" her if she went ahead with her plans to marry a man outside of her faith. Vi's family is Roman Catholic and her fiancé is Jewish. Initially, her boyfriend, David, said he was willing to convert to Catholicism, but decided against it when he met with resistance from his parents and asked if she was willing to convert to Judaism. Vi felt as though she could not bear the loss of her boyfriend, her parents, or her religion and slit her right wrist with a kitchen knife. Her mother found her and called 911; Vi was brought into the emergency department. She was operated on by a hand surgeon with the goal of full use of her right hand. Vi was then hospitalized for a week and a half in the inpatient mental health unit of the hospital.

Vi lives with her parents and has no siblings. Vi works as a bookkeeper for her father's furniture business. She has worked at this position since she graduated from high school. Vi did not go to college because it would have meant leaving her position at the store. Every time she mentions she is thinking of leaving the business, her father begs her not to leave or threatens to kick her out of the house and cut her off from any assistance. She may need to find and set up a new apartment.

Vi had rarely very little, and David is her first serious romantic relationship. He had worked at her father's store until the two started dating; he decided to quit to avoid the comments from Vi's father. The two had tentatively planned to marry in 6 months, but are now not sure what to do about the religion issue. Both sets of parents object strongly to the union. Vi still has close friends from high school, with whom she goes out a few times a month to movies, restaurants, and shopping. Vi loves to shop and find bargains. She enjoys manicures and pedicures and is usually dressed nicely. She exercises regularly at the gym, and David often joins her. She and David enjoy movies, cooking dinners at his apartment, and going on hikes with his dog. Vi's only goal is to get married to David, and if she cannot do that, then she does not want to continue living.

Lowenstein NA, Halloran P.
Case Studies Through the Health Care Continuum:
A Workbook for the Occupational Therapy Student, Second Edition (pp 155-157).
© 2015 SLACK Incorporated.

ANALYSIS OF OCCUPATIONAL PERFORMANCE

During her psychiatric stay, Vi was given a dorsal blocking splint, which she wore 24 hours a day. On orders from the physician, the charge nurse instructed the mental health workers to assist Vi in following a postsurgery modified Duran protocol that was to be carried out every hour. The protocol includes PROM flexion and extension to all joints, and use of the splint to protect the repair and promote movement. Vi exercised only if she was reminded to do so. Vi had no functional limitations before the suicide attempt. Since her discharge from the inpatient facility, she is scheduled to see a psychiatrist three times per week on an outpatient basis. This is her first time in counseling and first time on antidepressants. She had her sutures removed 2 weeks after the surgery. When she came to the outpatient department, it had been 2.5 weeks since the suicide attempt and resultant injury. She is scheduled to see the hand surgeon again in 3 days.

Upon OT evaluation, Vi exhibits no hearing, visual, sensory, or perceptual limitations. She responds to questions slowly, as if she has limited energy to answer. Her voice is soft and frail. Vi has no long-term memory deficits, but does display some difficulty with immediate recall and short-term memory. This appears to be due to a decreased attention span and inability to focus on the conversation.

Vi is left-handed. She has no physical limitations other than those related to the tendon laceration. Vi has active right digit extension as follows: 50 degrees metacarpophalangeal (MCP), –20 degrees proximal interphalangeal (PIP), and full distal interphalangeal (DIP) extension. Passively, she has 60 degrees MCP flexion and 40 degrees PIP flexion contractures beginning with the ability to move only half range to distal palmer crease. She has 30 degrees DIP flexion passively. Vi has slight edema in all digits, and the skin appears fragile and glossy. Vi denies pain or discomfort while wearing the splint. She reports doing her exercises faithfully, but it is apparent that this is not so.

Vi is independent in mobility. She reports independence in self-care and says the OT at the hospital taught her how to get dressed and wash with one hand. Vi says she has been doing almost everything that she had been before except cooking (due to lack of appetite), cleaning (due to disinterest), and working. Vi also reports not driving at this time. She states she simply avoids two-handed tasks and does things slowly with her left hand.

Vi wants to regain full use of her right hand so she "won't look like a freak." Vi says, unenthusiastically, that she will participate in OT as her doctor ordered. Her affect remains sad throughout the evaluation. Her next appointment for OT is set for the day after Vi's visit to the doctor.

QUESTIONS

Occupation

1. What occupations are most affected by Vi's injury to her hand? By her depression?

2. What occupations are least affected by Vi's injury to her hand? By her depression?

Performance Patterns

3. What roles have been most affected by Vi's injury and depression? How would you address these roles during your OT interventions? Is it appropriate to address roles in an outpatient clinic?

4. What routines have been most disrupted by Vi's injury and depression? How would you address this during your OT interventions?

Performance Skills

5. Identify 10 key performance skills that have been negatively affected by Vi's injury.

6. Identify 10 key performance skills that you identify as strengths that would assist during intervention.

7. How might you incorporate treatment of Vi's decreased attention span and recall into your hand therapy sessions?

8. Do you feel it is appropriate to address Vi's depression in outpatient OT? Why or why not?

Client Factors

9. Identify important values and beliefs that may influence your OT intervention.

10. Identify 10 body functions that are affected by Vi's injury. How might these affect her overall engagement in occupation?

11. What specific precautions should Vi follow to protect her tendon repair? What could happen if she does not follow these precautions? How could you reinforce Vi's adherence to precautions?

12. What issues might develop if Vi does not follow her exercise protocols?

13. How would you explain to Vi how to care for her dorsal blocking splint?

Contexts and Environment

14. Identify key personal and temporal contexts to consider for assessment and intervention.

15. Are there cultural contexts to consider during your assessment and intervention planning?

16. At what point do you think Vi will be physically and/or emotionally ready to return to her job? Explain your thinking.

17. If Vi were to return to work now, what type of accommodations would need to be made for her?

18. How might this injury have affected Vi's relationship with her parents?

19. What impact will the relationship with her parents have on Vi's progress?

20. How might this injury have affected Vi's relationship with her fiancé? What impact would that have on her progress?

21. How would you educate Vi's family about her injury and recovery process?

Theory and Evidence

22. What theory/theories or frame(s) of reference might you use in developing an intervention plan? Describe the rationale for your choice(s).

23. What, if any, evidence can you find to support your choice of theory/theories and/or frame(s) of reference?

24. What, if any, evidence can you find to support intervention?

Intervention Plan and Goals

25. What questions would you have for the hand surgeon before designing Vi's OT intervention plan?

26. Are there other standardized assessments that you would like to administer? What are these, and what information would you gain?

27. Write out a problem list for Vi.

28. What long-term goals would you and Vi set for OT intervention?

29. What short-term goals would you and Vi set for OT intervention?

30. If the hand surgeon orders active wrist flexion within the splint in addition to the present protocol, how would this change your intervention plan?

Situations

31. Vi's doctor now tells her that she is allowed active digit flexion within the splint. How would this change your intervention plan and goals?

32. Vi tells you that the only reason she wants to get her hand function back is so that she can use it to try to kill herself again. How do you respond to this?

33. Vi is minimally compliant with her exercises and home program. Why might this be?

34. Vi's father accompanies her to one of her OT sessions. He stands up and demands that you explain to him why his daughter is "not allowed" to return to work. What would you do?

35. Vi's father starts blaming you for her slow progress. His voice is escalating, and Vi starts to cry. What would you do?

36. How could you help improve Vi's follow-through with her home program?

37. Vi has cancelled the last two OT sessions. What would you do?

38. Vi's PIP contractures improve very little. What would be your course of action?

39. What might the hand surgeon decide to do at that point?

40. How might the hand surgeon's decision affect Vi's psychological status? Her physical status?

41. Vi tells you her father wants her to come back to work right away. She asks if you could explain her situation to him so he will not force her back too soon. What would you say to her in response?

Discharge Planning

42. Vi's progress is at a plateau. However, when you begin to speak of discharge, she promises to work harder. Explain your reaction to her promise. Describe what you would say to her, and what your next course of action would be.

43. What would your feelings be regarding Vi's discharge from therapy?

Financial Disclosures

Susan Gelfman has no financial or proprietary interest in the materials presented herein.

Patricia Halloran has no financial or proprietary interest in the materials presented herein.

Iris G. Leigh has not disclosed any relevant financial relationships.

Nancy A. Lowenstein has received payment for conducting workshops for the National Multiple Sclerosis Society.

Cathie Marqusee has no financial or proprietary interest in the materials presented herein.

Kathryn Prizio has not disclosed any relevant financial relationships.

Debra G. Sharp has no financial or proprietary interest in the materials presented herein.

Kimberly Witkowski has no financial or proprietary interest in the materials presented herein.

Index